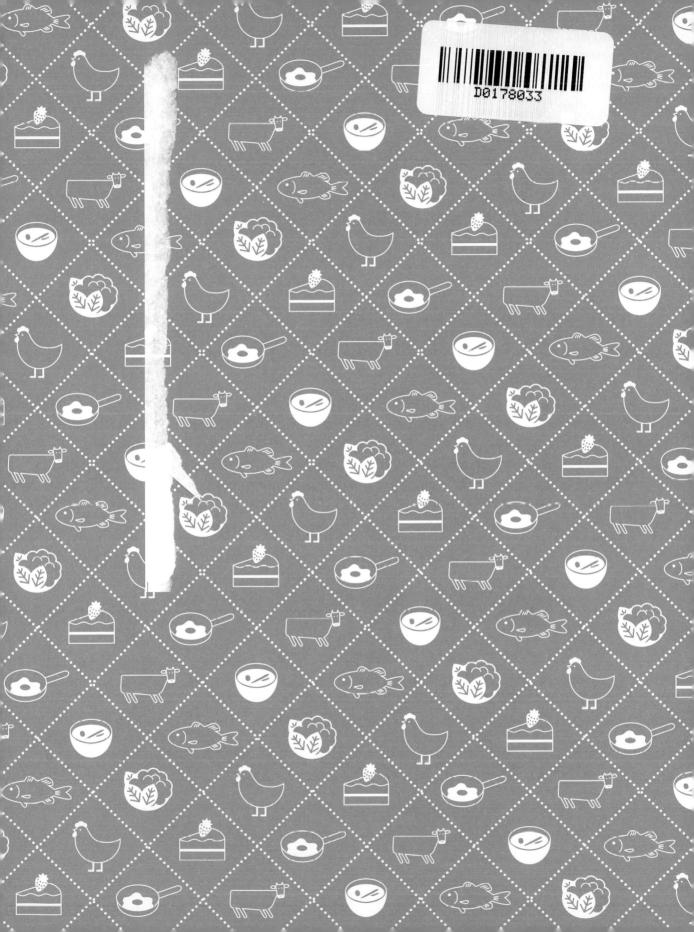

LOSE WEIGHT
FOR
GOOD

LOSE
WEIGHT
FOR
GOOD

Full-flavour cooking
for a low-calorie diet

TOM KERRIDGE

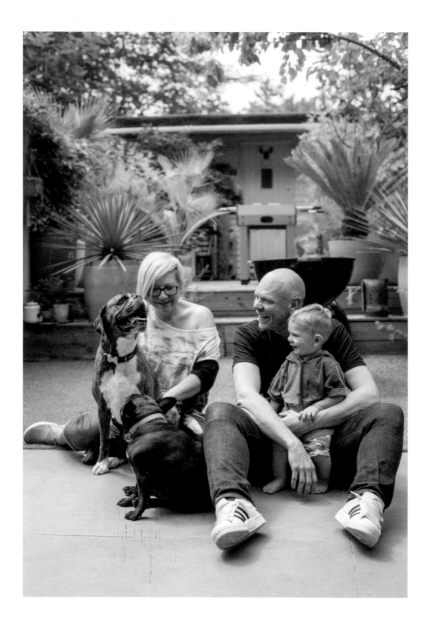

This book is dedicated to anyone who wants to, has to, or has already lost weight. It's all about the journey!

Big love and massive hugs to my 'everything', Bef, Acey and the daft dogs.

CONTENTS

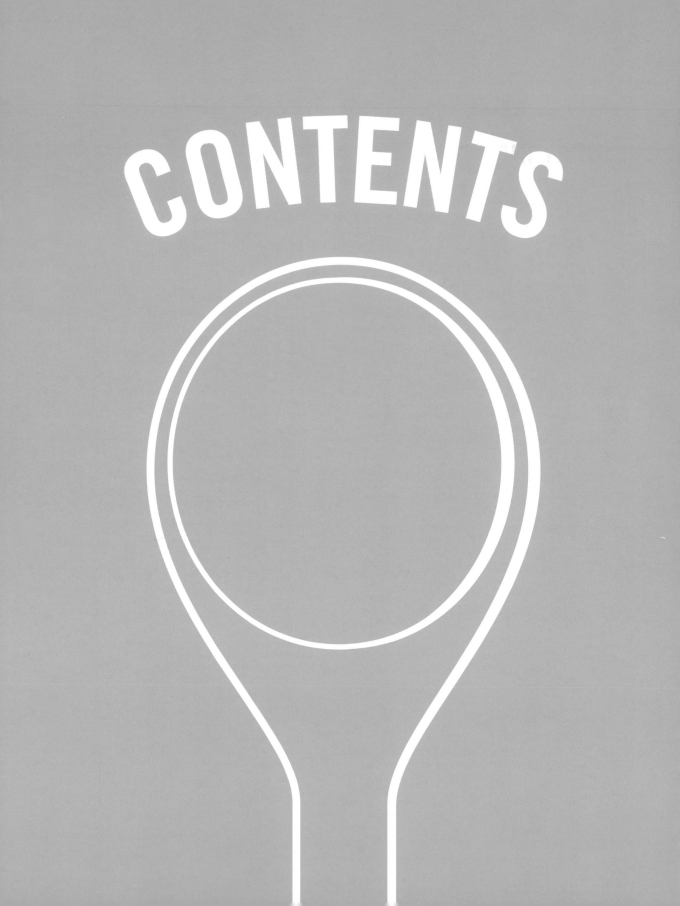

LOW-CALORIE DIETING.. 8

KEY INGREDIENTS.. 18

KIT LIST.. 23

BREAKFAST 28

SOUP 54

FISH & SEAFOOD.. 76

CHICKEN & TURKEY 104

MEAT 142

VEGGIE 178

SWEET THINGS 214

WEIGHING FRESH PRODUCE...................... 242

INDEX.. 245

A NOTE ON CALORIE COUNTS

The calorie counts for recipes cannot be absolutely precise because there are many variables, including the water and fat content of ingredients, and caloric loss during cooking (from draining off fat, for example). The counts do, however, allow you to roughly work out your daily calorie intake.

A NOTE ON OVEN SETTINGS

The oven timings in these recipes are for fan-assisted ovens. If you are using a conventional oven, you will need to raise the oven temperature by around 15°C. Ovens vary, so use an oven thermometer to verify the temperature and check your dish towards the end of the suggested cooking time.

LOW-CALORIE DIETING

To lose weight we know that we need to eat less and move more. We are told by doctors, nutritionists, dieticians and personal trainers that it's all about a balanced diet and eating fewer calories than we use. There's plenty of good advice out there, so why are so many people in Britain still overweight?

I think bland and unappetising 'diet food' is a major factor. How can you stick to a diet if you're not enjoying the food? If lower calorie food came packed with flavour and in generous portions, people would be more likely to lose weight. And this is where I believe I can help, by providing lots of delicious and satisfying recipes that are also lower in calories. I want to help more people to lose weight for good – regardless of lifestyle and skills in the kitchen – without ever scrimping on flavour.

It's no secret that I used to be a big lad! At my heaviest I weighed in at around 30 stone and my health was suffering. When I celebrated my fortieth birthday, I knew I had to make a change, and fast, or else I might not get to see my fiftieth – or my little boy grow up. Things were that serious.

As a chef I am surrounded by food all day and I wasn't going to give that up. I lost weight by cutting down drastically on carbohydrates: potatoes, pasta, bread and rice. It meant I could carry on tasting the food I was working with every day in the kitchen while still cutting back on what I ate. And it worked for me – I've lost 12 stone and I'm still going – but I understand that this isn't the best approach for everyone.

A calorie-restricted diet, where you consume only a certain amount of calories – based on your height, weight-loss goals and the amount of exercise you do – is much easier for many people to stick to because you can still eat many of your favourite foods, as long as you don't go over your daily limit. (You can talk to your GP about calculating the number of calories you should have each day, or use one of the reliable calculators online to estimate this yourself.)

I realise that counting calories is a bit boring. But soon you'll get to know the calories in the ingredients you use regularly so you won't have to think about it so much. And as for the recipes in this book, all the counting has been done for you!

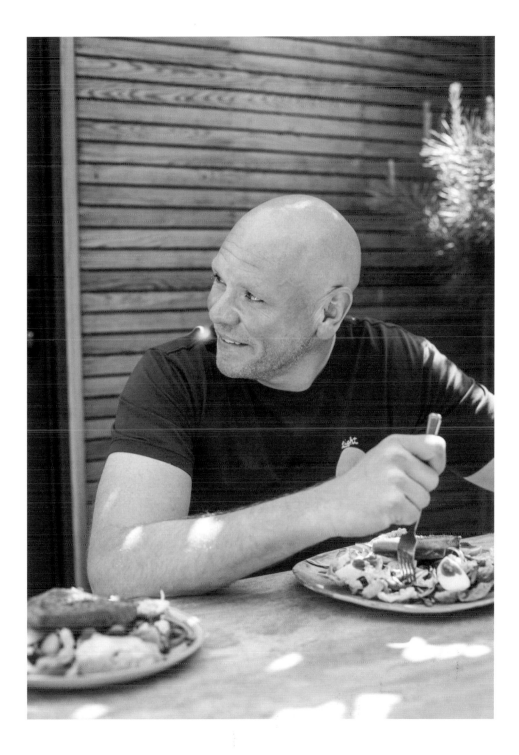

SO WHAT CAN I EAT?

When you're on a diet, especially one where you're reducing your calories, it's all too easy to focus on what you can't eat and what you think you'll be missing out on. Food is one of the biggest pleasures in life as well as one of the most important factors in our health, and we just won't succeed if we stop enjoying it.

The beauty of a lower calorie diet is that you can still eat many of the foods you love, as long as you don't go over your daily limit. Obviously, if you were to eat a massive fry-up for breakfast with a stack of toast, you would need to drastically restrict your calories for the rest of the day, but in theory it would be possible.

If you like bread, rice, pasta and potatoes, you can still enjoy them. Many calorie-controlled diets seem to reduce the portions of your regular foods right down. So, yes, you may be eating steak with a blue cheese sauce or chocolate brownies but the servings will be tiny! You'll be hungry, craving something more. I'm all about creating bigger portions, as the secret to dieting success is to feel satisfied and full.

So now for the fun bit: let's focus on great food and what you can eat! And let's make this the driving force for a new way of eating. My recipes are designed to achieve satisfyingly large portion sizes, that have extra layers of flavour and plenty of interesting textures to keep your meals exciting. Hopefully this will ease the journey that you are about to embark on.

I use a lot of fresh herbs and spices, garlic and chilli, as they provide huge flavour for virtually no calories. I also sometimes include a small amount of a high-flavour, higher calorie ingredient, such as smoked salmon or cheese. You don't need much of these strongly flavoured ingredients to make an impact and stop you feeling like you're missing out.

Texture is just as important. Chefs use fats to help get both flavour and texture into their cooking, but if you're cutting out the fats you need to find other ways of getting flavour and texture onto your plate. I have some clever techniques to help you out here. Try to balance crunchy ingredients – like fresh, healthy veg – with something creamy. Pair spicy heat with salty or cooling flavours, and acidity with sweetness. If you can get the right balance, it doesn't matter how few calories the dish contains, it will taste great.

As a general rule, I don't like the idea of replacing regular ingredients with lower calorie alternatives – they are often flavourless poor imitations and I'd rather just use something else entirely. But there are a few low-cal options that I do use in these recipes, as they can be an easy and subtle way to cut back on calories. Cooking spray oil, which has just one calorie per spray, can really drop the overall

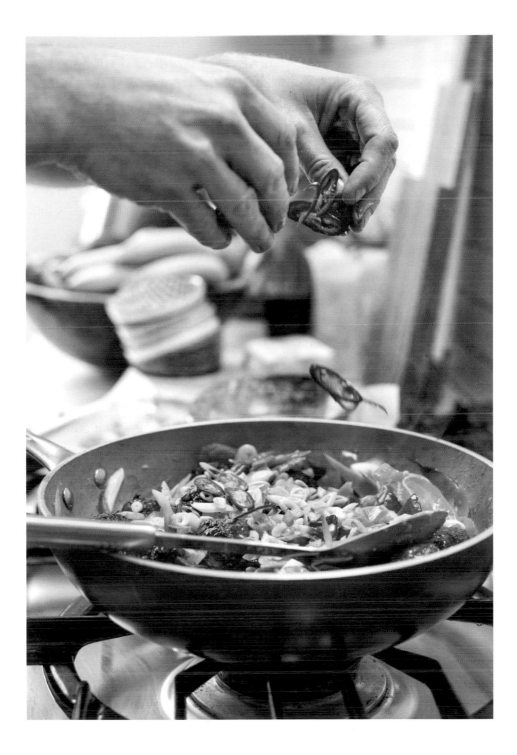

count. And a swirl of reduced-fat cream replacement stirred through soups or puddings adds a satisfying richness that low-calorie diets often lack. I also use a sugar replacement to add a bit of sweetness where needed. Reduced-fat pastry is a great addition to the shopping list too. Although losing weight is all about shifting your mindset and getting rid of old unhealthy habits, we can have the occasional treat, and a crispy fruit tart may tick all the boxes.

GETTING CLEVER IN THE KITCHEN

As we lead increasingly busy lives, being faced with complicated dishes that take ages to plan and cook is a recipe for diet failure. I want to show you how to make everyday food that is incredibly simple and totally delicious. Lots of the recipes in this book can be made in less than half an hour, and most can be made ahead in part, or full, and frozen, too. It's all about maximum flavour for minimum effort.

Favourite recipes often taste so good because they use lots of butter and/or oil to roast or fry the ingredients to caramelised perfection. I'll show you some easy techniques that will create tasty effects like these without adding calories. You'll find a cook's blowtorch a handy investment for giving a dish those lovely crispy browned edges you usually get from roasting or frying. It may sound a bit cheffy but it's an easy way to add flavour, and create extra texture for zero calories.

Something as simple as roasting mince before you use it adds a huge amount of extra flavour and texture – try it in my One-layer lasagne (page 152). A regular, go-to ingredient for dieters is chicken, as it is high in protein yet low in fat, but it can shrink or dry out when you cook it, leaving you feeling disappointed. I poach chicken crowns on the bone in some of my recipes, which helps the chicken keep its volume – upping the portion size (surely every dieter's dream) while also keeping the meat lovely and moist. Try it and see what a big difference it makes to the finished dish in my healthy version of Chicken tikka masala (page 122).

Cooking low and slow in the oven is another great way of ensuring meat stays succulent and keeps its flavour without adding lots of oil. This method works brilliantly with casseroles and pot-roasts, but I also use it for roasting a whole chicken. Next Sunday, instead of your usual roast, give my Piri piri chicken on page 136 or Pot-roast topside of beef (page 156) a go.

A classic dieter's downfall is to pile up a healthy salad and then smother it in a high-fat oily or mayo-loaded dressing. Suddenly your sensible choice can have as many calories as a takeaway! To solve this little dieting dilemma, I've come up with a clever oil-free dressing, using a little cornflour to give it a thick consistency – you would never think it was virtually calorie-free. You can flavour it in different ways to give an instant hit to salads and veg, or drizzle the dressing over meat or fish – try the smoked paprika version on page 183, the herby option on page 186 or the citrus dressing on page 152.

Just a few simple adjustments to the way you prepare and cook your food can save a huge amount of calories. In fact, I'd go as far as to say that many of these dishes have ended up tasting better than the meals they were created to replace, because they have so much more flavour and texture.

DON'T BE BEATEN BY A POTATO!

Even armed with good advice and tons of tasty recipes, no one can say losing weight will be easy. Dieting is hard. Everyone wants to carry on eating burgers and drinking at the weekend, and lose weight at the same time, but you can't!

You really have to want to do it, it's as simple as that. If you find yourself raiding the fridge at 3am the only person you have to answer to is you. But I know that when you've got some entrenched habits, changing the way you eat is tough.

For many, it involves a huge lifestyle change and you have to be committed. When you're a healthy weight and have an active lifestyle you can afford to have the odd day when you eat more calories than you need and it will balance itself out overall. But when you need to lose weight, you have to commit to lower calories every day. And it's not just for the 12 weeks or 6 months of your 'diet' either, it's about changing your whole mindset for good. Once you've lost that 2 stone – or 10 stone! – you can't just go back to the way you were eating before. I used to smoke like a chimney but cutting down to 10-a-day still made me a smoker and it's the same with food: you have to change the whole way you think about what you eat.

When you have a large amount of weight to lose, it can be hard to believe you will ever make it to your goal. But after just a week or two of eating only the amount of calories you actually need, you really will lose weight. And once you start to see those changes, it will make it so much easier to keep going.

Getting comfortable with a diet or any new habit and sticking to it is all about routine. Exercise is just one routine, eating regularly and well is another. It will help you stay away from bad food choices because you will feel in control of your life and able to make good decisions.

I totally get it though; I had loads of days when I found it a real struggle – especially surrounded by all that delicious food. But what helped carry me through – and resist temptation – was remembering the reason that I wanted to lose weight in the first place.

For me, the main motivations were my son and my health. Losing weight meant I'd be able to have a kick about with him in the park and have a better chance of being around for him as he got older. Work out what your main motivation is and whenever you feel yourself weakening, picture it in your mind. Maybe even cut out a photo of something that reminds you of your goal or reason for keeping to your diet and stick it in your wallet – or on the fridge!

There are a few little tricks that I still use today, which really help me keep my focus. Try them out and see if they help you:

1. Think of a hero of yours. Mine are mostly sports-related but it can be anyone you think has achieved something amazing. They will have made a commitment to get to the top and sacrificed a lot on the way; it didn't happen overnight. You can be your own hero! But you have to give up some things to reach where you want to be. And you might have to be a little bit selfish about it. Do what you need to do to get results.

2. Now remember a time in your life when you accomplished something you really wanted. Remember how difficult it was to get there? Then remember how amazing you felt when you did it. You've done it before so you can do it again. Imagine how brilliant it will feel when you reach your weight-loss goal. Think of what you can achieve if you set your mind to it.

3. This might sound strange, but it can also help to turn food into animated characters in your head. If you're tempted to eat some crisps or a bag of chips, imagine a potato with a face on it. Now arm wrestle with it! You wouldn't let the potato win would you? Don't be beaten by a potato!

4. This is a bit more serious, but when I'm feeling like I'm going to give into cravings, I think of people less fortunate than me all around the world. It puts things into perspective in an instant. Why am I worrying about a chocolate bar? Other people have it far worse than me.

It's been shown that losing weight with other people can be more effective than going it alone. Finding someone to give you a few words of praise or a kick up the bum when you need it can make the difference between success and failure. I've been so impressed by the support I've seen people give each other through their ups and downs. Maybe pair up with a mate, or a group of dieters, and keep in regular contact. You can reach out to them when you need a boost – they'll know what you're going through. Meet up for a cup of tea (without the slice of cake) or a walk in the park. It can help to know that you're not on your own.

The support of those around you every day is also key to dieting success, so make sure everyone knows what you're doing and aiming to achieve. Get your partner and kids on board. Ultimately, it's going to be up to you to make good choices, but it can help knowing that everyone wants you to succeed.

And then there's the obvious way to help prevent you reaching for the snacks: if you don't go filling your house with crisps, chocolate bars and ice cream then you'll be less likely to eat them. It can really be as simple as that!

GET ORGANISED

Often, convenience foods aren't healthy. To stay on track you need to be organised and make your diet work for you. With the best will in the world, if it's dinner time and you're starving when you are halfway up the motorway it's going to be harder to make a healthy choice when faced with what's on offer at the service station. Keeping in control of what you are eating when you're out of the house is often a problem for dieters, and planning ahead and being prepared are the answers.

I remember my mum sending me off to school with my favourite packed lunch – corned beef and mustard sandwiches in an old plastic box. (I was well jealous of the boy in my class who came in with a new Superman lunchbox.) Invest in some good plastic containers. They are cheap to buy and those mini thermal flasks are brilliant too for winter warmers like soups and stews. There are lots of easy recipes in this book that are ideal for when you're out and about – including the soups on pages 58–63 and 66–9. You'll make your workmates jealous!

But if you haven't packed yourself a lunch, calories are printed on most packaging now, so you can check and still make a good choice. Go somewhere where you can read the labels so you know exactly what your meal contains.

Something as simple as using a smaller plate can help trick your mind into thinking you've eaten more – the plates we use nowadays are *huge* compared to the plates our grandparents ate from. It's no wonder our portion sizes have got a bit out of control. And try to stick to three meals a day. Snacking is where it often goes wrong! That's why it's important to keep portion sizes reasonably big, without going overboard. Most of the time we're not even hungry when we reach for a snack, it's just a habit we've got into, so learn to recognise if you really are hungry or you've just got used to that chocolate biscuit with your afternoon cup of tea.

I heard about something recently called 'the broccoli test': if you had to replace your snack of choice with a piece of broccoli, would you still eat it? If not, then you don't need it! And if you do need a snack to keep you going, get used to eating fruit. My go-to snack is cold grapes straight from the fridge.

Being on a diet doesn't mean you should enjoy your meals any less; in fact, enjoying what you eat can really help you stick with it. Set the table, light a candle, do whatever it takes to make mealtimes feel special – no more mindless eating in front of the TV. If you're at the table you'll pay much more attention to what you're actually eating, which will make you feel more satisfied by it.

There's nothing better than sharing a meal with your friends and family – it's what brings us together – and you shouldn't have to miss out just because you're trying to lose weight. But a lot of people worry about what to do when they eat out. It can often feel like dieting will have a negative impact on your social life, especially as you'll probably be cutting out the booze at the same time.

Most restaurants now offer healthier options on their menus and some give the calorie content too. Pick one of these if you can. Many menus are online now, so you can choose in advance, which means you're less likely to be swayed by anyone else when you get there. If they don't have any obvious lower calorie options, then just ask. The kitchen team and front of house staff want happy customers and they deal with different needs all the time so it's really no big deal to make something lower calorie. Be brave and ask them to help you. Perhaps they can grill a piece of meat or fish and serve it with some salad. Also remember you're among friends. Tell them what you're doing and that you want them to support you, and I'm sure they will. Stay strong and you'll come away having had a great evening, knowing you haven't undone all your good work.

A FINAL NOTE

If you've been carrying a bit of extra weight around for a while then you may feel as though it's become part of your identity – it's just part of who you are. I've been called 'Big Tom' for most of my adult life. I still am, even after losing 12 stone! I think some big guys and girls worry they'll lose a part of themselves if they shed the weight. But surely being healthy is a better badge of honour than being big?

Once you've lost a few pounds, you'll start to feel good. And this will help you carry on towards your weight-loss goal. There's also the little boost that comes when you can fit into your old clothes again – or maybe buy some new ones.

Be a good example to others and inspire them to follow a new, healthier lifestyle like you. You can show them it is possible!

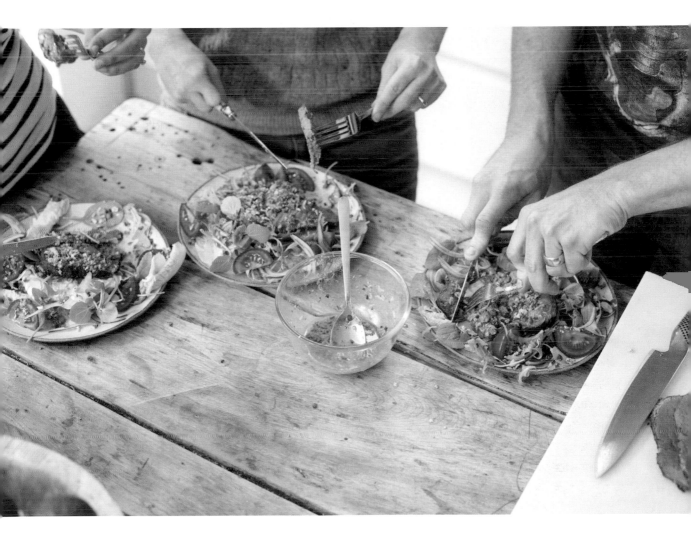

KEY INGREDIENTS

When you are on a diet, every mealtime should be about maximising flavour, texture and portion size, so you feel full and satisfied and never feel like you're missing out. These are some of my favourite ingredients that won't pile up the calories but will still deliver on taste.

Cauliflower 'rice' You can buy this in packets, but it is preferable – and easy – to make your own by grating cauliflower on a box grater or in a food processor. If you use it instead of regular rice (or mix the two together), you'll be full from the extra fibre and you can have a larger portion size as the cauliflower version has virtually no calories.

Chicken This is a popular dieter's choice, as it's low in fat but high in protein. In some of my recipes I use chicken crowns, which are cooked with the breasts still on the bone – this helps the meat to keep its size and stay succulent as it cooks. You can, of course, use regular chicken breasts or thighs instead, but a crown will give a better result.

Chickpeas and beans High in protein and fibre, these are handy to have in the cupboard for instantly bulking up soups, stews and curries. I like black beans, butter beans, kidney beans and mixed beans.

Chilli, garlic and ginger I use a lot of these aromatics, as they pack a massive flavour punch for almost zero calories.

Cornflour This is effective for thickening sauces, and takes away the need for lots of flour, butter or potato. It's also a key ingredient in my oil-free dressings (see pages 152, 183 and 186). It's important to mix cornflour to a smooth paste with a little water before adding it to the dish, as you don't want clumps of unmixed cornflour in there.

Cream alternatives Reduced-fat substitutes for single and double cream, often labelled 'light single (or double) cream alternative', are useful if you're on a diet. These are made from a blend of buttermilk and vegetable oils, to be lower in calories than real cream but provide a similar rich taste and consistency.

Dairy reduced/low-fat options Skimmed or semi-skimmed milk, reduced-fat cheese, 0% fat yoghurt, quark, ricotta and low-fat spreads are easy lower calorie swaps. In particular, 0% fat Greek yoghurt has a thick and creamy texture so it can easily replace higher calorie foods, such as cream, crème fraîche, soured cream and mayonnaise. It has no fat but is high in protein and is filling, with a tangy taste. Quark is a lesser known low-fat cheese curd and is great for making cheesy-tasting dishes – and cheesecakes, like the one on page 231.

Eggs Always use organic and free-range eggs if you can. Eggs are great to have on hand for a quick low-cal meal.

Fish and seafood These are a great source of low-fat protein. Fresh is best, so get to know your fishmonger and find out when the fish is delivered. Salmon and other oily fish may be higher in calories than white fish, but they're a great source of valuable omega-3s and really good for you. Keep a bag of frozen prawns in the freezer and a tin of good-quality tuna in the cupboard for meals that can be assembled in minutes.

Fruit If you need to snack, eat fruit. Opt for varieties that are lower in sugar and calories, like berries and apples. Lemons and limes are flavour powerhouses – buy them unwaxed and use both the zest and juice when cooking. The natural sweetness of fruit means you can make it the basis for your puddings too.

Herbs Fresh coriander, mint, basil, thyme (including lemon thyme), chives and flat-leaf parsley will introduce fantastic layers of flavour and extra texture to your cooking. Dried herbs are stronger in flavour than fresh ones, so you won't need to use as much.

High-flavour, higher calorie ingredients Using just a small amount of ingredients such as smoked salmon, Parma ham, chorizo, cheese, truffle oil, sesame oil, coconut milk, chocolate, nuts and seeds can boost your mealtimes. You don't need a lot of these rich ingredients to make a meal feel really special. Just watch your portion control!

Hot sauce and mustard These offer an instant way of adding extra flavour to a recipe. I like to add a spoonful of mustard to marinades and stews, and I'll drizzle hot sauce over just about anything.

Meat Always buy the best meat you can afford, preferably free-range and grass-fed – check with your butcher. Opt for lower-fat cuts, such as tenderloin, lamb leg or lean mince (5–10% fat) and trim off any visible excess fat where you can. Before roasting or cooking meat, take it out of the fridge and allow it to come up to room temperature, loosely covered, on the work surface. The closer the meat is to its final eating temperature, the more evenly it will cook. And don't forget to rest your meat once it is cooked, for extra tenderness.

Pastry, pre-rolled reduced-fat There is nothing wrong with using ready-made puff pastry! Even most chefs have this to hand because making your own takes ages. You can get reduced-fat options now, usually with around 30% less fat. Filo pastry is another excellent way of adding crunch when you're in need of something a bit special.

Salt and pepper A properly seasoned dish can make all the difference between bland food and a tasty, satisfying meal. I generally use flaky sea salt and freshly ground black pepper. For Asian-style dishes, I usually rely on soy sauce for seasoning. If you are looking to lower your salt intake, you can, of course, use less in the recipes and reduced-salt soy sauce where appropriate.

Spices An easy shortcut to maxing out flavour for virtually no calories is using spices. I use them in rubs and marinades for meat, as well as in curries and all manner of spicy dishes. The ones I use most often are ground cumin, ground coriander, turmeric, paprika (hot and smoked), dried chilli flakes, cardamom, Chinese five-spice and ground mixed spice. Toasting spices in a dry pan before you use them – or letting them cook for 30 seconds or so before you add the other ingredients – can really intensify their flavour. Spice pastes such as harissa, chipotle and curry paste are great to have on standby too, to add instant interest to meat or vegetables. Spices are also thought to help curb your appetite!

Spray oil At just one calorie a spray this will instantly cut down on all the calories you usually add with regular cooking oils and fats. Both olive oil and sunflower oil versions are available.

Stock If you're making any of the chicken crown recipes in the Chicken & Turkey chapter (pages 104–141), you'll have lots of fresh chicken stock in your freezer. Always try to use fresh stock (including veg and fish stock) whenever you can,

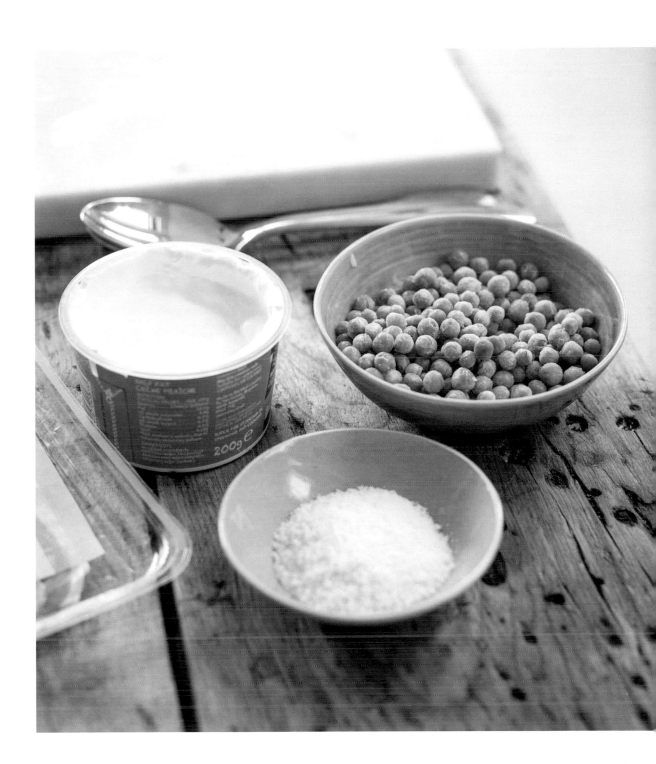

as it makes such a difference to the finished dish. You can buy fresh stock in most supermarkets. Otherwise, use a really good stock cube.

Sweeteners I have used a sweetener in place of regular sugar in some recipes to cut back on calories (most sweeteners are virtually calorie-free). I mostly use erythritol, although inulin is a good option if you're looking to caramelise it. Stevia is becoming very popular now, but just be aware that it can be a lot sweeter than other sweeteners. I also use agave syrup (from the agave plant) in a few recipes, which is a bit like honey or maple syrup but it has a sweeter taste so you only need to use a little. In the long term, it will help your weight loss if you can adjust to preferring a less sweet taste, so try to reduce the amount of sweetener you add to dishes over time.

Sweets, biscuits and crisps NO! You can't lose weight and carry on eating the way you were before. Forget about these unhealthy, high-calorie snacks that were doing you no good at all. If you're eating proper, satisfying meals, you won't even want them. Remember: don't be beaten by a potato!

Tortillas Corn, wholewheat and wholegrain tortillas are higher in fibre than plain flour tortillas, keeping you fuller for longer. Keep a pack of tortillas in your freezer for quick and easy wraps, burritos and pizza bases. I also use them for making tacos (see page 172).

Turkey mince This low-fat mince makes a great alternative to beef or lamb mince. Just remember that it can dry out more quickly than regular mince as it cooks, so keep it moist with lots of extra veg.

Vegetables Most veg are low in calories and packed with nutrients and fibre, so using more of them is an easy way to reduce the overall calorie count of your meals. Substantial veg like aubergines and mushrooms are good alternatives to meat, and they're lower in calories than potatoes. A tub of dried mushrooms is a particularly useful store-cupboard standby. Swap regular white potatoes for sweet potatoes or celeriac (this makes a great mash); both are lower in starch and higher in fibre, so they'll fill you up. And make sure you eat your greens too – I love broccoli, kale, cabbage and courgettes. Shredded cabbage and spiralized courgettes are brilliant alternatives to pasta. Frozen peas are great to have on hand in the freezer, and tins of tomatoes are essential.

KIT LIST

If you're cutting back on calories, there are some simple cooking methods that will optimise flavour. It's worth investing in a few items of equipment that make your life easier and your mealtimes more satisfying.

Blender or food processor These make light work of soups and sauces. A food processor is useful for really working flavours into ingredients, for example when you're making my Lamb doner (see page 162). It's also handy for whizzing up cauliflower into 'rice'.

Cook's blowtorch I know this sounds a bit cheffy, but you can get a decent cook's blowtorch quite cheaply and it offers an easy way to create those delicious, sticky, caramelised and charred effects and the smoky flavours you usually only achieve by roasting or frying food in lots of cooking fat or oil. Blowtorching is also a very useful way of searing meat without frying it, or adding crunch to your ingredients. To use a blowtorch safely, don't touch the flame and always check the gas has been switched off when you finish. Place the food on a metal tray before you start and make sure there is no flammable material, such as alcohol, nearby. Always light the blowtorch before putting it near raw food, or you run the risk of getting fuel on the food. The best technique is to use a sweeping motion, where the flame waves slowly back and forth across the surface to evenly 'scorch' the food. Don't concentrate too long on one area, or the food may burn.

Deep-lipped baking tray This is really useful for when you're pre-roasting mince, which I often do. You can break up and turn the mince over as it cooks and if the meat releases any juices as it cooks (turkey mince is likely to do this) then they won't spill into your oven.

Graters A micro or fine grater is a must for grating lemon zest, garlic and ginger. A larger box grater is best for grating carrots, courgettes and other veg. Grating ingredients makes them go further, so you won't need to eat as much.

Griddle pan Using one of these will give meat and vegetables a lovely charred effect, as in Griddled veg and halloumi with couscous (page 186), but you can just use a normal frying pan instead.

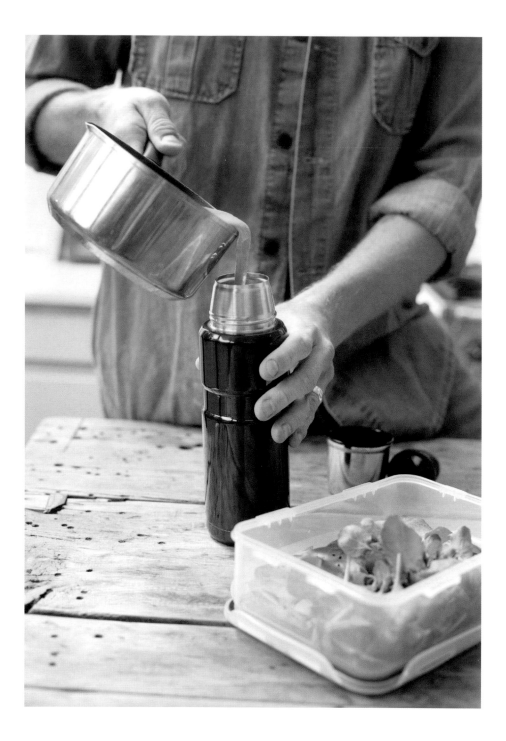

Muffin tray Muffins are a handy breakfast choice when you're short on time, and you'll need a muffin tray to bake them in. I also use a muffin tray to make 'tacos' (see page 172).

Non-stick pans A good non-stick frying pan and large saucepan will cut down the need for oil when you're frying.

Spiralizer I can't stop talking about how great these are! Spiralizers are basically a glammed-up version of a veg peeler. You can turn courgettes into courgetti – a brilliant low-calorie alternative to pasta that actually tastes of something, unlike the original spaghetti. You can also spiralize cucumbers and firm fruit and veg, such as apples, carrots and squashes.

Thermal flask and food storage containers Sticking to a diet is all about thinking ahead and being prepared. Invest in some good freezer storage containers so you can freeze portions of soup and make extra batches of meals to stash in the freezer. No excuses for reaching for the takeaway menu! Most of the meals in this book can be packed up and taken to work for lunch too. A flask is great for soup, making dieting in the winter months a whole lot easier.

Thermometers (oven and meat) It's worth making sure your oven is at the correct temperature before you start cooking, which you can check by placing an oven thermometer on the middle shelf. It is consistently hotter near the top, where the main heating element is positioned, so as a general rule, if you need something to brown well on the surface, such as a gratin, put it on an upper shelf in the oven. Some of my recipes involve cooking meat for a long time at a lower temperature than usual, so I recommend you also get a meat thermometer to check that your meat is properly cooked through.

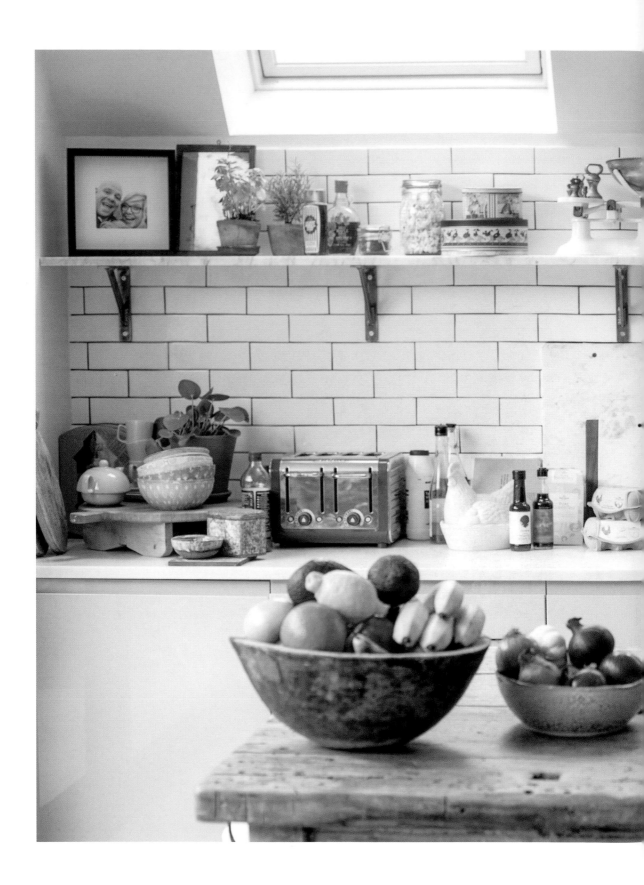

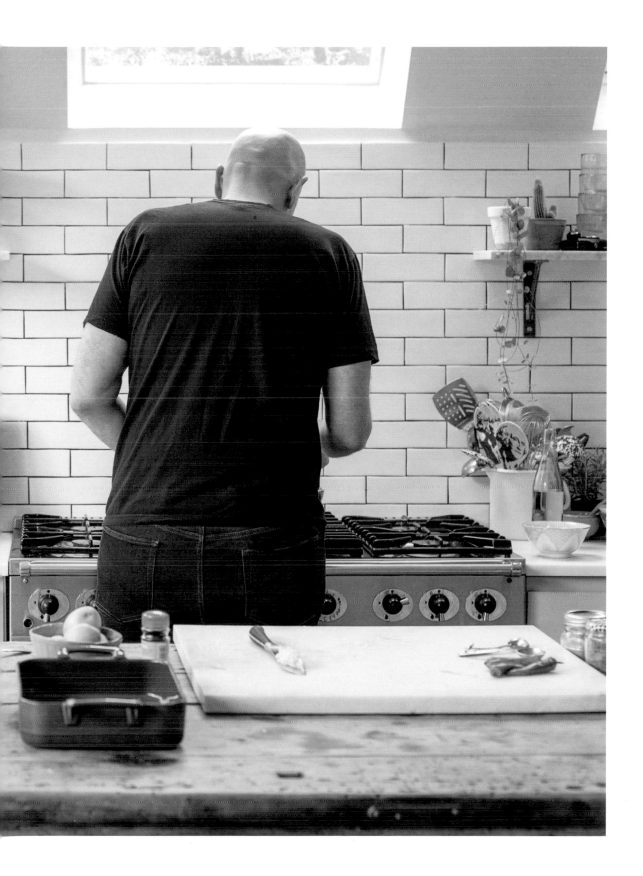

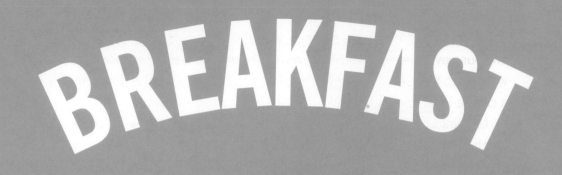

BREAKFAST

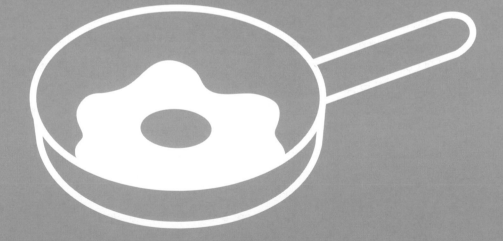

We all know that breakfast is the most important meal of the day, and that's true even when you're watching your weight. If you don't eat something first thing, you'll be thinking about food all morning and counting down the minutes to lunch. And if you happen to walk past a bakery on your way to work, you'll find it so much harder to resist those delicious smells wafting up the road – before you know it, you'll be through the door and buying a calorie-laden pastry. So make sure you eat a proper breakfast!

Mornings are often busy, but if you sit down to eat breakfast, as you would lunch or dinner, you'll feel so much more satisfied – my Blueberry, lemon and thyme pancakes (page 33) are really easy to whip up and the Bircher muesli on page 36 can be made the night before.

If you're used to eating a bowl of sugary cereal every morning then it can take a while to adjust to less sweet breakfast dishes. But packaged sugary cereals are doing you no good, so ditch them! Eggs are great for breakfast, as they are low in calories but full of nutrients. Smoked ham and courgette tortilla (page 51) is one of my favourite ways to start the day; it's also perfect for a packed lunch and tastes great the next day too.

If you have a bit more time in the morning, then give the Shakshuka eggs on page 44 a go. It's a brilliant healthy breakfast, with loads of protein from the eggs and warming spices – a fantastic sharing brunch dish for the weekend.

But even when you're organised, sometimes life just gets in the way. For days like these, have a batch of Apple and raisin or Apricot and cranberry muffins (pages 30 and 40) at the ready and grab one as you head out the door. They are full of contrasting flavours and textures to keep things interesting – with the added bonus of getting some extra fruit in there.

If you really are caught out, then there are other low-cal options you can turn to. Even a slice of toast with reduced-fat spread is better than nothing. Yoghurt is a great choice (just watch the sugar content in low-fat options), maybe with some fruit on the side. If you like something a bit sweeter in the morning, my Puffed rice cereal with banana and date yoghurt (page 39) is delicious.

Start the day well and you're more likely to stick with your diet. All it takes is a little planning ahead to keep you on the road to achieving your weight-loss goals.

Apple and raisin muffins

These muffins are brilliant to have ready to go for those mornings when you're rushing out the door. The Chinese five-spice and sesame oil lend a great savoury edge to the traditional flavour combination of apples, raisins and honey, and the oats on top give them a satisfying crunchy finish.

Makes: 12

Calories: 190 per muffin

3 tbsp runny honey
2 medium Braeburn apples, peeled and diced
1 tsp Chinese five-spice powder
1 tsp ground mixed spice
2 large free-range eggs, beaten
3 tbsp toasted sesame oil
200ml semi-skimmed milk
2 small bananas, peeled and mashed
300g self-raising flour
2–3 tsp granulated sweetener
1 tsp bicarbonate of soda
40g raisins

For the crumble topping
1 tbsp rolled oats
1 tbsp light brown sugar

THE LOWDOWN Caramelising the honey first gives these spiced fruity muffins an extra, rich layer of flavour.

1. Preheat the oven to fan 180°C/gas 4. Line a 12-cup muffin tray with large muffin cases.

2. Put the honey into a small non-stick saucepan over a medium heat and heat for 2–3 minutes to caramelise gently, until it turns a dark golden brown and just begins to smoke. Add the apples, along with the spices, and stir gently for 3–4 minutes or until slightly softened. Remove from the heat and leave to cool.

3. Combine the beaten eggs, sesame oil and milk in a bowl. Mix in the mashed bananas.

4. In a large bowl, stir together the flour, sweetener, bicarbonate of soda and raisins. Make a well in the middle. Pour in the egg mixture and add the apples with any liquid from the pan. Stir gently to combine.

5. Spoon the mixture into the muffin cases. Mix the oats and sugar together and sprinkle on top of each muffin. Bake on the middle shelf of the oven for 20 minutes. To test, insert a skewer into the centre: it should come out clean. If not give them a few minutes longer.

6. Leave the muffins to cool a little on a wire rack, then eat while still warm. They will keep for up to 3 days in a tin and can be reheated in an oven preheated to fan 160°C/gas 3 for 5 minutes.

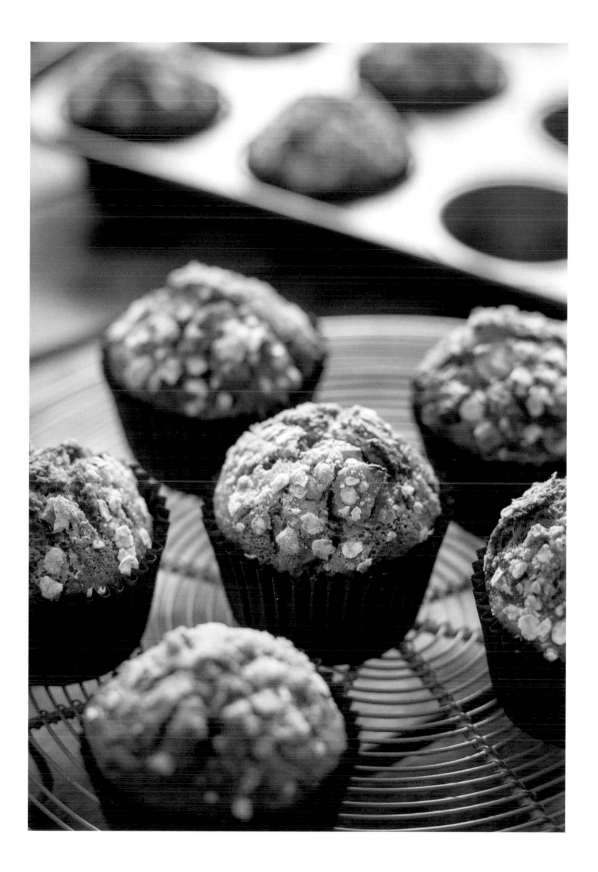

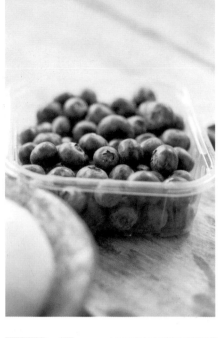

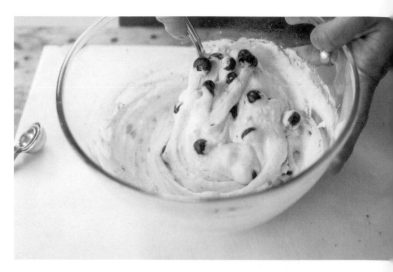

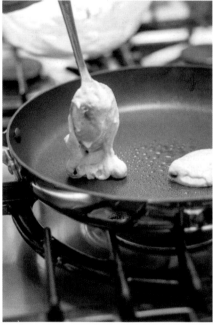

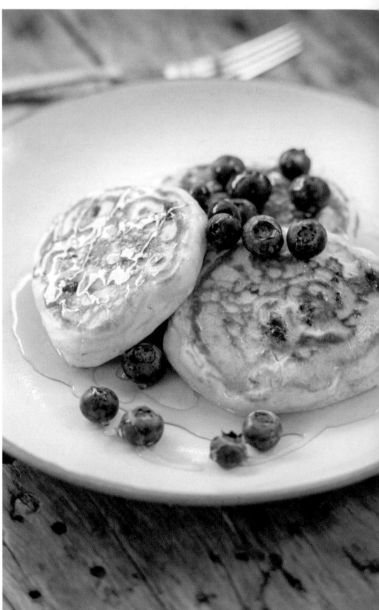

Blueberry, lemon and thyme pancakes

Pancakes are a real treat for breakfast, yet they are so easy to knock up in the morning. These include ricotta, which is a great dairy product to use when you are on a diet as it's low in fat but still rich and creamy. Lemon thyme brings the fresh flavours together.

Serves: 4

Calories: 300 per serving

200g plain flour
1 tsp cream of tartar
1 tsp bicarbonate of soda
2–3 tsp granulated sweetener
1 tsp lemon thyme leaves,
    chopped
Finely grated zest of 1 lemon
175ml semi-skimmed milk
1 large free-range egg
50g ricotta
200g blueberries
Sunflower oil spray
2 tbsp agave

1. Combine the flour, cream of tartar, bicarbonate of soda, sweetener, thyme leaves and lemon zest in a large bowl and make a well in the middle.

2. In a jug, whisk together the milk, egg and ricotta. Pour into the well in the flour mixture, then whisk until you have a thick, smooth pouring batter. Fold in half of the blueberries.

3. Heat a non-stick frying pan over a medium heat and add a few sprays of oil. Spoon 3 dollops of batter into the pan to form 3 pancakes. Cook for 3 minutes on each side, then remove from the pan. Keep warm, wrapped in foil, while you cook the remaining pancakes.

4. Serve 3 pancakes each, scattered with the remaining blueberries and drizzled with agave.

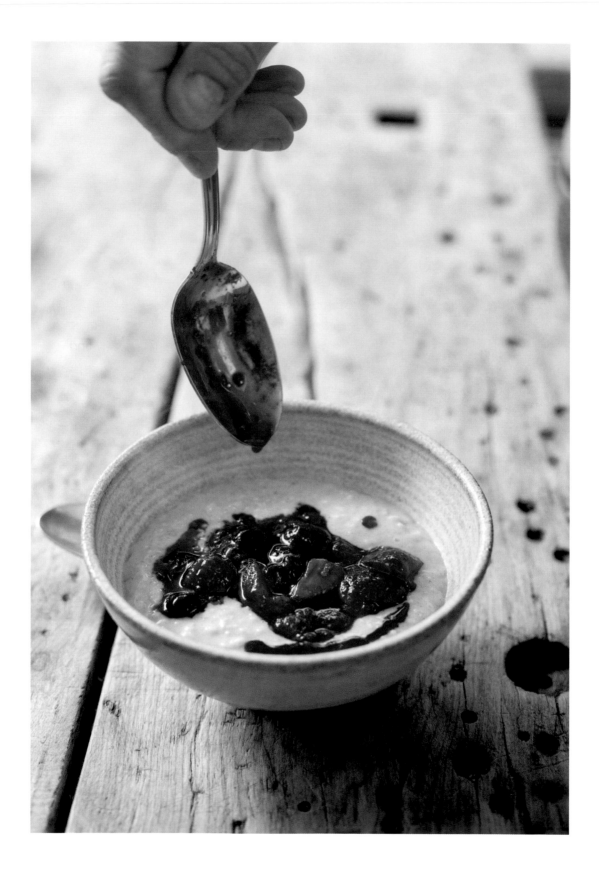

Overnight porridge with berry compote

As much as we're meant to enjoy it because it's so good for us, porridge can sometimes be a bit bland. This warm mixed berry compote brings it to life – a bit like swirling jam through your rice pudding as a kid…

Serves: 4
Calories: 290 per serving

160g jumbo rolled oats
600ml semi-skimmed milk
300ml water
1 tsp ground cinnamon
1 vanilla pod, split and
    seeds scraped
1–2 tbsp granulated sweetener

For the berry compote
350g mixed berries (strawberries,
    blueberries and raspberries)
2 tbsp maple syrup
1 tbsp water

1. Place the oats, milk, water, cinnamon and vanilla seeds in a bowl. Stir well and chill in the fridge overnight.

2. The following day, transfer the mixture to a non-stick saucepan and place over a medium heat. Stir in the sweetener and bring to a simmer. Cook, stirring occasionally, for 8–10 minutes or until the oats are cooked and the porridge is lovely and creamy. If it gets too thick, add some boiling water.

3. Meanwhile, prepare the berry compote. Halve or quarter the strawberries, depending on size. Put them into a small pan with the other berries, the maple syrup and water. Bring to a gentle simmer and cook for 5 minutes then remove from the heat.

4. When the porridge is cooked, divide it between four bowls and top with the warm berry compote. Serve immediately.

THE LOWDOWN Oats release their energy slowly, helping to sustain you for longer so you're less likely to feel the need for a snack mid-morning.

Blueberry and apple Bircher muesli

A bowlful of this delicious, sustaining muesli will see you through to lunchtime. Apples, almonds, toasted fennel seeds and honey give it lots of character and baking the oats and nuts first lends a lovely, toasty flavour.

Serves: 2
Calories: 440 per serving

60g rolled oats
2 tbsp flaked almonds
1 tsp fennel seeds, toasted and
    crushed
150g natural yoghurt (0% fat)
100ml skimmed milk
100ml fresh apple juice
1 tsp granulated sweetener
2 large or 3 small eating apples,
    peeled and grated
60g blueberries
2 tsp runny honey, to serve

1. Preheat the oven to fan 180°C/gas 4.

2. Spread out the oats on a baking tray and toast in the oven for 10–15 minutes, until starting to turn golden brown and a little crunchy. Set aside to cool on their tray.

3. Place the almonds on another small baking tray and toast in the oven for 5–6 minutes or until they are very brown – this will give your Bircher a deep nutty flavour. Set aside.

4. Place the cooled oats in a medium bowl and sprinkle over the crushed toasted fennel seeds. Stir in 100g of the yoghurt, the skimmed milk, apple juice, sweetener and grated apples. Mix well and leave in the fridge for a minimum of 3 hours, or overnight.

5. The next morning, stir through the remaining yoghurt. Divide between bowls and sprinkle with the toasted almonds. Top with the blueberries and drizzle over a little honey to serve.

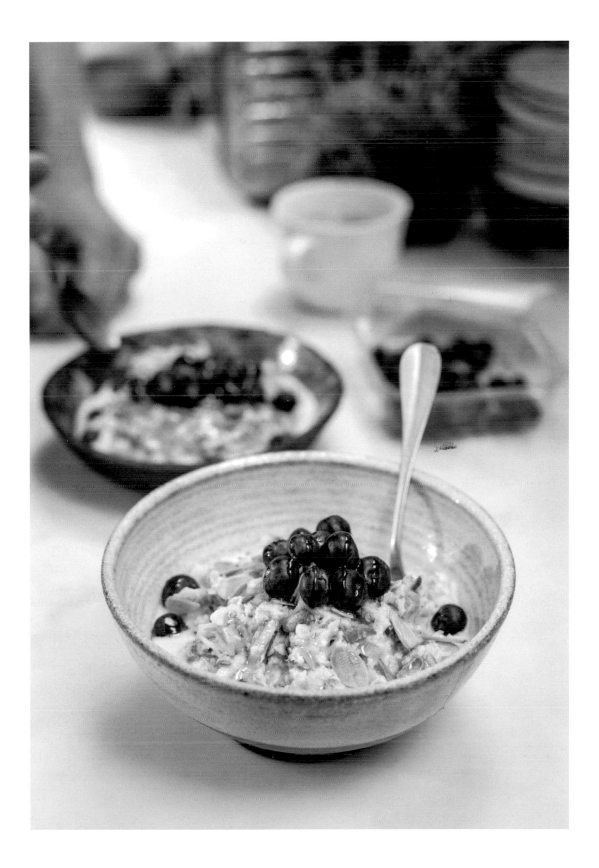

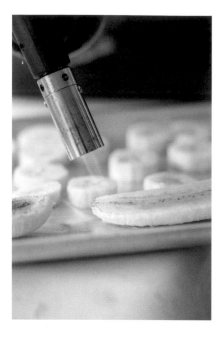

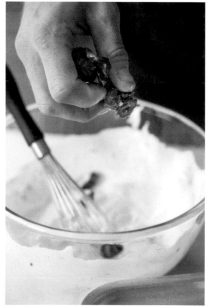

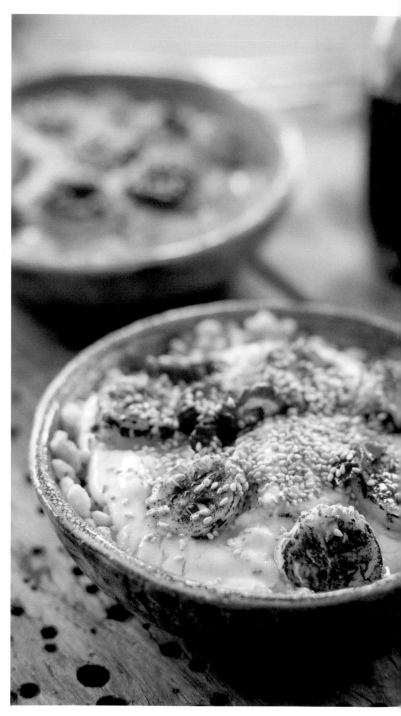

Puffed rice cereal with banana and date yoghurt

Dates are a great natural alternative if you're used to sugary breakfast cereals in the morning, but they are quite high in calories so don't get carried away! The crispy, crunchy texture from the puffed rice and sesame seeds combined with the sweet, smoky caramelised bananas makes this a really satisfying breakfast.

Serves: 2

Calories: 400 per serving

2 medium bananas, peeled
20g puffed rice cereal
200g natural yoghurt (0% fat)
100g Greek yoghurt (0% fat)
4 medjool dates, pitted and
    sliced
1 tbsp maple syrup
2 tsp sesame seeds, toasted

1. Slice one banana lengthways and place, cut side up, on a baking tray. Slice the other banana into thick rounds and lay these on the same tray. Using a cook's blowtorch, caramelise the uppermost surfaces until brown and charred. Roughly chop the halved banana.

2. Divide the cereal between two serving bowls.

3. Whisk the two yoghurts together. Stir the roughly chopped banana, half of the dates and 1 tsp maple syrup into the yoghurt.

4. Spoon the yoghurt over the cereal and top with the slices of banana and remaining dates. Sprinkle with sesame seeds and trickle over the rest of the maple syrup.

THE LOWDOWN I often sprinkle toasted seeds onto a bowl of yoghurt and fruit to add flavour and crunch. Toast the seeds in a dry frying pan for a minute or so until golden and fragrant, shaking the pan to make sure they colour evenly. Toasted seeds are great scattered over salads and soups too.

Apricot and cranberry muffins

Dried cranberries are one of my favourite ingredients to use because they have a fantastic level of acidity that helps cut through any sweetness. Using mashed bananas is a good butter replacement, keeping things creamy, while the orange adds a fresh, zesty flavour. The crunchy coconut topping provides a great contrasting finish.

Makes: 12

Calories: 170 per muffin

1 large, very ripe banana, peeled
200ml skimmed milk
3 tbsp sunflower oil
2 large free-range eggs, beaten
Finely grated zest and juice of
    1 orange
250g self-raising flour
2 tbsp soft light brown sugar
2 tbsp granulated sweetener
1 tsp bicarbonate of soda
½ tsp ground ginger
1 vanilla pod, split and
    seeds scraped
50g dried apricots, chopped
30g dried cranberries

For the topping
1 tbsp desiccated coconut
1 tbsp rolled oats

1. Preheat the oven to fan 180°C/gas 4. Line a 12-cup muffin tray with large muffin cases.

2. In a bowl, mash the banana well with a fork. Add the milk, oil, eggs and orange zest. Measure out 4 tbsp of the orange juice and add to the bowl. Mix well.

3. In a separate large bowl, mix together the flour, brown sugar, sweetener, bicarbonate of soda, ginger, vanilla seeds and dried fruit. Add the banana mixture and mix until just combined.

4. Divide the mixture between the muffin cases and sprinkle the desiccated coconut and rolled oats on top. Bake on the middle shelf of the oven for 15–20 minutes, until the muffins are golden on top and firm to the touch.

5. Allow the muffins to cool a little on a wire rack, then eat while still warm. They will keep for up to 3 days in a tin and you can reheat them in an oven preheated to fan 160°C/gas 3 for 5 minutes.

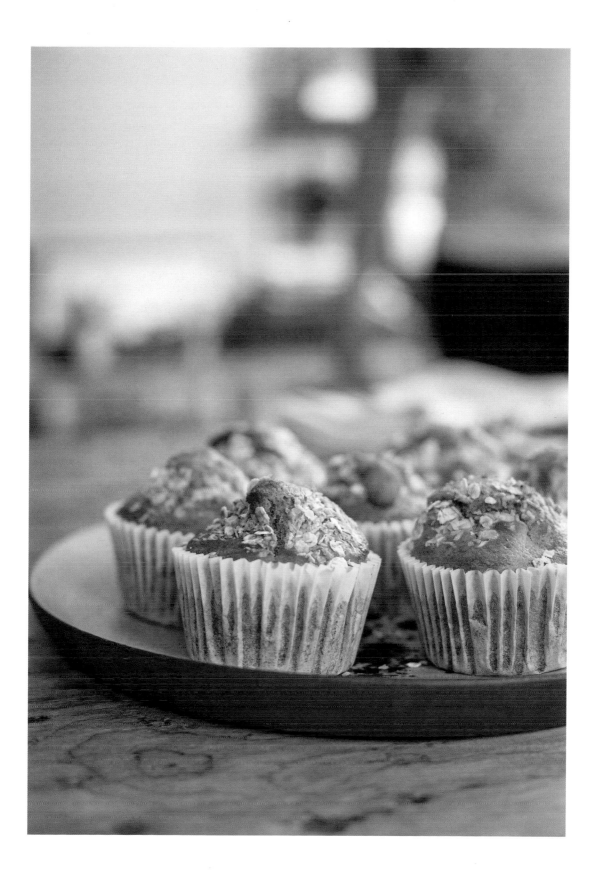

Baked doughnuts with sweet five-spice dust

Doughnuts, on a diet?! Yes, it is possible, if you bake them instead of frying them, replace some of the fat in the batter with semi-skimmed milk and add a little spice to the usual all-sugar coating to max out the taste and lessen the calories. A real treat of a breakfast!

Makes: 12

Calories: 120 per doughnut

180ml semi-skimmed milk
25g butter
1 tsp fast-action dried yeast
250g self-raising flour
1 tsp baking powder
2 tbsp granulated sweetener
½ tsp sea salt
½ tsp ground cinnamon
½ tsp Chinese five-spice powder
1 large free-range egg, beaten
Sunflower oil spray

For the five-spice dust
40g golden caster sugar
½ tsp Chinese five-spice powder

1. Pour the milk into a small saucepan. Add the butter and place over a low heat until the milk is just warm. Remove from the heat and leave until the butter has melted. Stir to combine, then whisk in the yeast.

2. Mix the flour, baking powder, sweetener, salt, cinnamon and Chinese five-spice together in a large bowl. Make a well in the middle and pour in the warm milk mix and beaten egg. Using a wooden spoon, beat well to make a smooth, thick batter. Transfer to a large piping bag.

3. Spray two 6-hole non-stick metal doughnut trays with about 12 sprays of oil in total. Snip the top off the piping bag and pipe the batter into the moulds to half-fill them. Leave to rise for 1 hour.

4. Preheat the oven to fan 210°C/Gas 6–7. Once the doughnuts have risen, cook them on the top shelf of the oven for 9–10 minutes until browned.

5. Meanwhile, mix together the ingredients for the five-spice powder dust and transfer to a small plate.

6. When the doughnuts are cooked, leave to cool slightly in the tin, then remove. If some of the holes have closed over in the oven, trim them to open up with a sharp knife.

7. Brush each doughnut with a little water and then dip the brushed side into the five-spice dust. Enjoy while they are still warm.

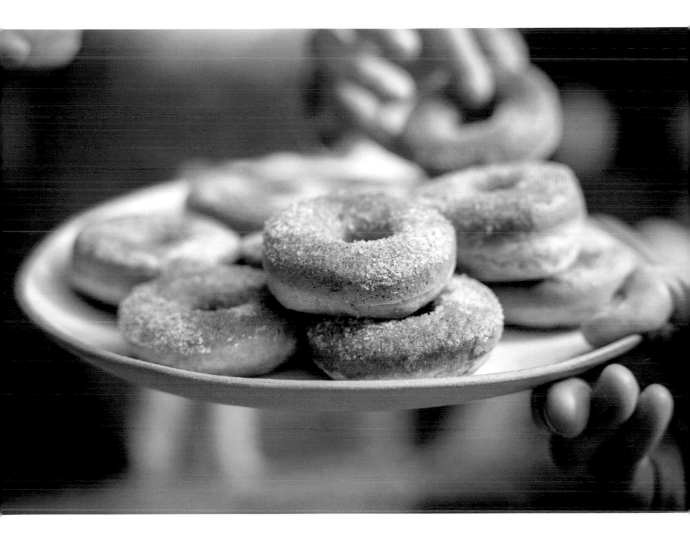

Shakshuka breakfast eggs

These easy Moroccan-style eggs, poached in a spiced tomato sauce, have become hugely popular. Make them and you'll be the most fashionable dieter in the country right now! The sauce is cooled by the deliciously salty feta crumbled on top.

Serves: 2
Calories: 375 per serving

1 tsp light olive oil
1 red onion, finely sliced
1 large red pepper, cored, deseeded and diced
1 large green pepper, cored, deseeded and diced
4 garlic cloves, finely sliced
1 tsp ground cumin
½ tsp ground cinnamon
2 tsp hot smoked paprika
A pinch of flaky sea salt
2 x 400g tins chopped tomatoes
4 medium free-range eggs
50g half-fat feta
A handful of coriander leaves, roughly chopped
Freshly ground black pepper

1. Heat the oil in a medium non-stick frying pan (that has a lid) over a high heat. Add the onion and cook for 2 minutes, then add the peppers and garlic and cook for a further 4 minutes. If the veg begin to stick, add a splash of water to the pan.

2. Stir in the cumin, cinnamon, paprika and salt and cook, stirring, for about 30 seconds, until the spices become fragrant. Tip in the tinned tomatoes, stir to combine and lower the heat. Simmer for 10–15 minutes until the sauce thickens slightly.

3. Make 4 small wells in the tomato sauce for your eggs. Crack an egg into each well and place a lid on top of the frying pan. Leave the eggs to cook for 5 minutes or until the whites are just set.

4. Crumble the feta over the surface and finish with the chopped coriander and a grinding of pepper. Serve straight from the pan.

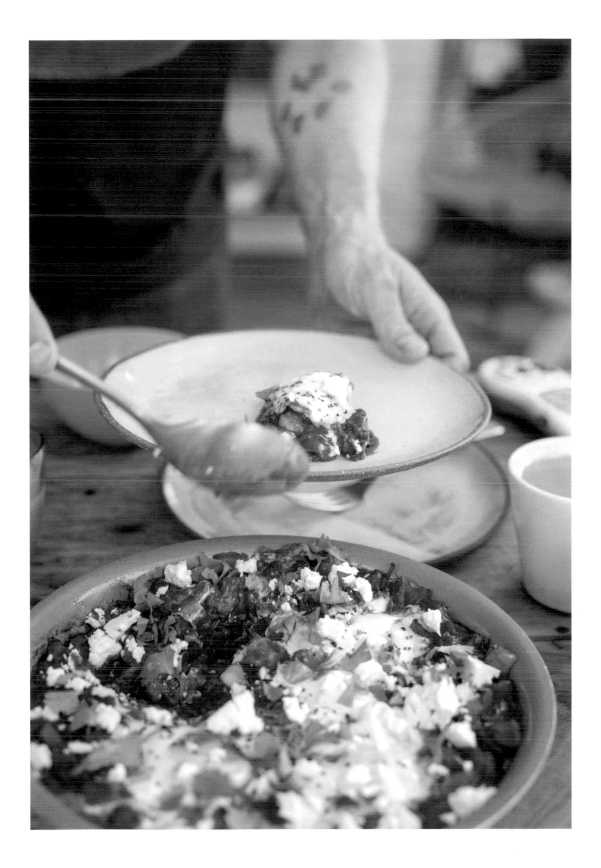

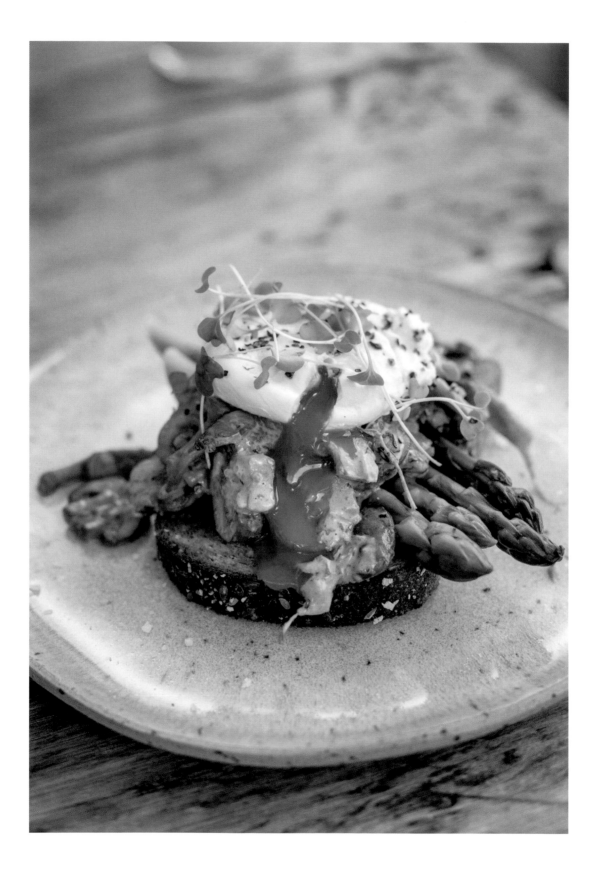

Creamy mushrooms, poached egg and asparagus

Big, punchy mushroom flavours are enhanced with a little porcini and truffle paste in this decadent brunch dish. The cream alternative adds a silky smooth richness so it won't feel like you're on a diet at all. It's also good without the toast for a lower calorie option.

Serves: 2

Calories: 265 per serving
170 without toast

1 tbsp half-fat margarine
2 garlic cloves, finely chopped
150g chestnut mushrooms, thickly sliced
100g oyster mushrooms, roughly torn
8 asparagus spears, woody ends trimmed and lower part of spears peeled
2 medium free-range eggs
1 tsp thyme leaves
1 tsp liquid aminos
1 tsp porcini and truffle paste
2 tbsp light single cream alternative
2 tbsp flat-leaf parsley leaves, finely chopped
Sea salt and freshly ground black pepper

To serve
2 slices of granary bread, freshly toasted
Salad cress or micro-cress, to finish

1. Heat a medium non-stick frying pan over a high heat and add the margarine. Once it has melted, add the garlic and both types of mushroom and cook, stirring frequently, for 4–5 minutes or until the mushrooms begin to soften and brown.

2. Meanwhile, add the asparagus spears to a pan of boiling salted water and simmer for 2–3 minutes until tender. Remove with tongs, drain and set aside; keep warm.

3. Stir the boiling water to create a whirlpool and crack in the eggs, one at a time. Poach at a simmer for 2–3 minutes until the egg whites are set and the yolks are still runny.

4. While the eggs are poaching, stir the thyme, liquid aminos and porcini and truffle paste into the mushrooms and cook for 1 minute. Stir through the 'cream' and chopped parsley, then taste and season with a little salt and pepper, if needed.

5. Place a slice of hot toast on each serving plate, lay the asparagus spears on top and spoon on the mushrooms. Using a slotted spoon, drain each poached egg (as soon as it is ready) and place on the mushrooms. Sprinkle with a little seasoning and scatter with cress to serve.

Scrambled Cajun eggs with spinach and kale

This dish is packed full of protein and slow-release energy to get you through to lunchtime. Cajun spice ramps up the flavour and you can serve it with hot sauce for an extra kick. For a bigger weekend breakfast, you could add grilled tomatoes or mushrooms on the side.

Serves: 2
Calories: 310 per serving

4 large free-range eggs
75ml light single cream
    alternative
Sunflower oil spray
½ red onion, diced
1 large green pepper, cored,
    deseeded and diced
40g kale, shredded
1 tbsp Cajun spice mix
A handful of spinach leaves (50g)
Sea salt and freshly ground
    black pepper
Hot sauce, to serve (optional)

1. Crack the eggs into a bowl, add the 'cream' and season well with salt and pepper. Whisk to combine.

2. Add 6 sprays of oil to a large non-stick frying pan and place over a medium heat. Add the onion and green pepper and cook for 3–4 minutes, until slightly softened.

3. Add the kale along with a splash of water and cook for 2 minutes. Now add the Cajun spice mix, a pinch of salt and the spinach. Cook, stirring, for about a minute, until the spinach has wilted.

4. Add another 6 sprays of oil to the pan. Pour in the whisked eggs and leave them to set for a few seconds, then gently stir them around until they are just cooked. You want them to remain soft and silky, so don't overcook.

5. Spoon the spicy mixture onto warmed serving plates. If you like it extra spicy, add a good dash of your favourite hot sauce.

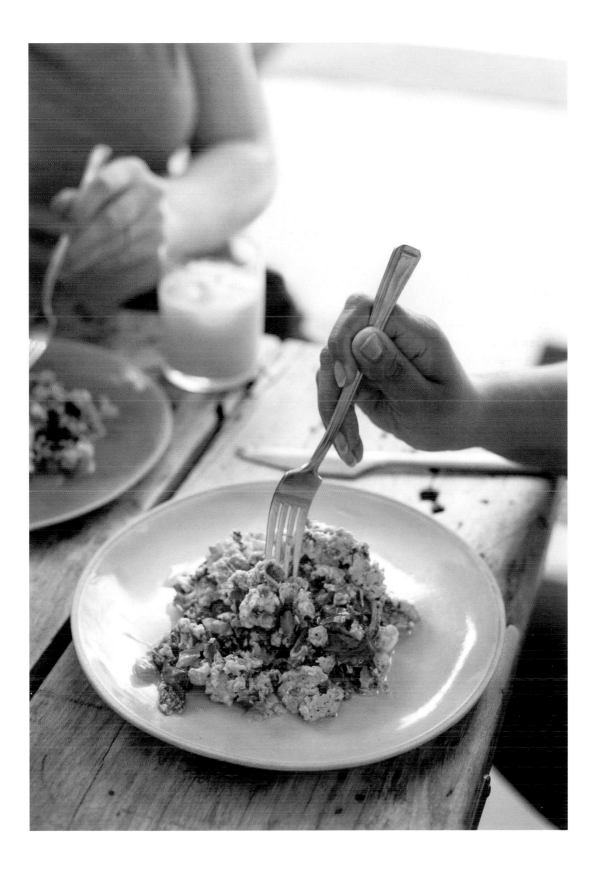

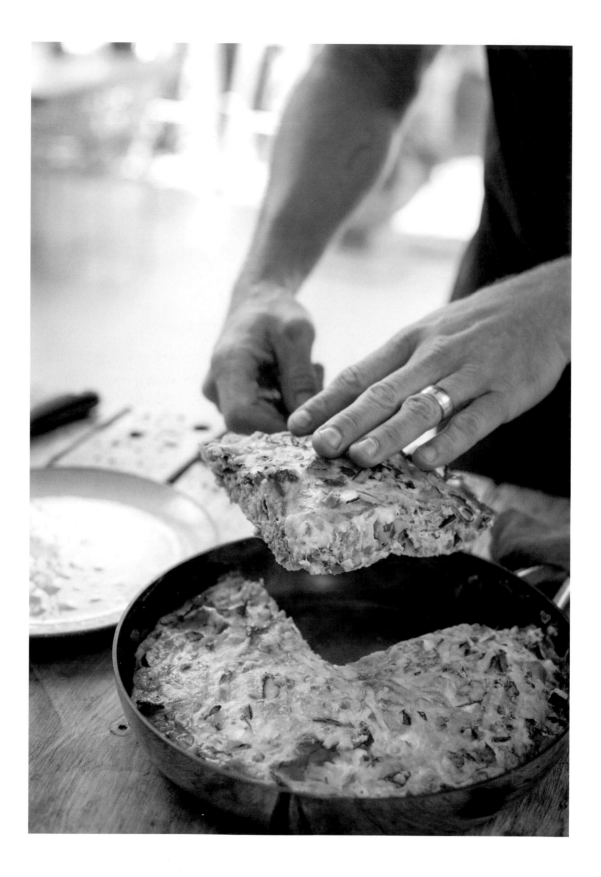

Smoked ham and courgette tortilla

Perfect hot or cold, you can even pack this breakfast up to eat on the go. It also makes a great lunch if you have any left over. Play around with the veg to suit your tastes – and what you have in the fridge. Diced peppers, chopped red onion, courgettes, tomato and roasted aubergine all work well.

Serves: 4

Calories: 345 per serving

Olive oil spray
2 small courgettes, diced
8 large free-range eggs
1 tsp Dijon mustard
2 tbsp light single cream
    alternative
A small handful of basil leaves,
    finely chopped
A small handful of flat-leaf parsley
    leaves, finely chopped
150g frozen peas
4 spring onions, sliced
200g thinly sliced smoked ham,
    roughly chopped
50g half-fat Cheddar, grated
Sea salt and freshly ground
    black pepper

1. Heat a 24cm ovenproof non-stick frying pan over a medium heat and spray with 10 sprays of oil. Add the courgettes and cook for 4–5 minutes or until just starting to brown. Remove from the pan and set aside.

2. Preheat the grill to medium-high.

3. Crack all the eggs into a large bowl and add the mustard, 'cream' and some salt and pepper. Whisk to combine, then mix in the basil, parsley, peas and spring onions.

4. Return the frying pan to a medium heat and add another 10–15 sprays of oil. Add the ham and cook for 2 minutes, then add the courgettes and mix through. Pour in the egg mixture and move it around with a rubber spatula until it begins to set.

5. Sprinkle the grated cheese over the surface of the tortilla and place under the grill for 5–7 minutes, until the cheese is golden and bubbling. The tortilla will have puffed up a little too.

6. Leave to stand for a few minutes, then loosen the tortilla from the sides of the pan, using a rubber spatula. Cut into wedges and serve, while still warm.

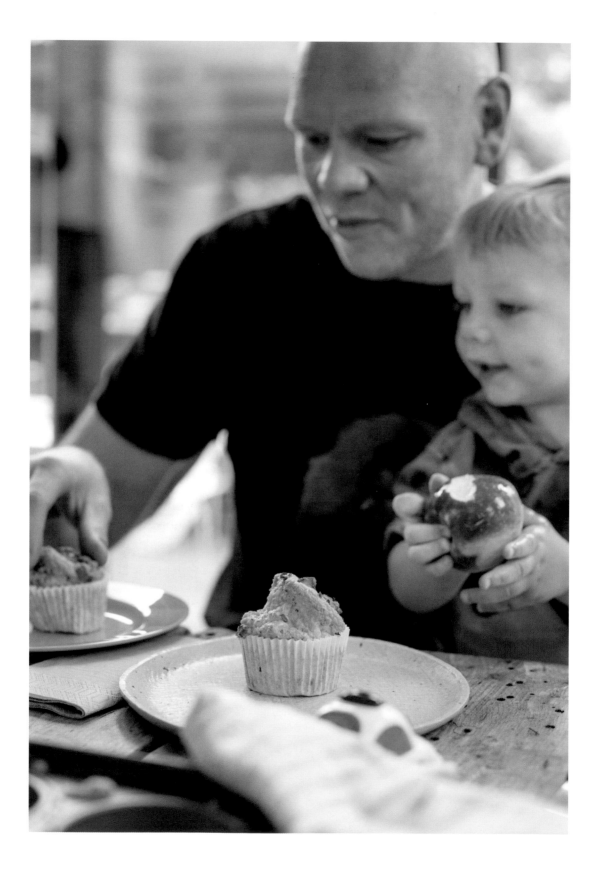

Salmon, egg and feta 'muffins'

These can be eaten hot or cold so they're ideal – and quick – to make the day before and stash in the fridge overnight. You get a huge amount of flavour from a very small amount of smoked salmon, so you don't need to use a lot to make these flour-free muffins feel really indulgent.

Makes: 9
Calories: 105 per 'muffin'

Olive oil spray
100g smoked salmon,
    cut into strips
2 spring onions, sliced
75g frozen peas
3 tbsp finely chopped chives
6 large free-range eggs, separated
75g half-fat feta, crumbled
Freshly ground black pepper

1. Preheat the oven to fan 180°C/gas 4. Place large muffin cases in 9 holes of a muffin tray. Spray each one with a few sprays of oil.

2. Put the smoked salmon, spring onions, peas and 2 tbsp of the chives into a medium bowl. Add the egg yolks and mix together.

3. Whisk the egg whites in a large, clean bowl until soft peaks form, then fold into the salmon mixture until evenly combined. Season with pepper and fold through 50g of the crumbled feta.

4. Divide the mixture between the muffin cases – it will come right up to the top of each case.

5. Carefully place the tray on the middle shelf of the oven and bake for 7 minutes. Crumble over the remaining 25g feta and 1 tbsp chives then return to the oven for a further 7–9 minutes, or until just set.

6. Sprinkle with a little extra freshly ground pepper and serve warm or cold.

. . . .

THE LOWDOWN If you use small amounts of luxury ingredients, like smoked salmon and feta, you won't feel as though you're restricting yourself by eating 'diet food'. Just watch your portion control.

. . . .

SOUP

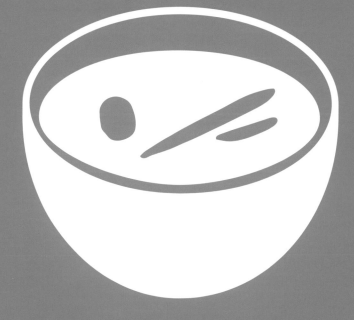

S oup is a godsend when you're on a diet, but I sometimes think that it gets a bad rap. Many people seem to think soup can be a bit boring – but that's only if you're eating a boring soup! The recipes in this chapter are all so delicious and varied there will be no chance of you giving in to cravings, even when you're away from home. Invest in a thermal flask and you can take your soup with you on the go.

Like any other food, soup should be about flavour and texture, and big portion sizes. My Asian Tom yum soup (page 65) is packed full of spicy aromatics and tons of crunchy veg, but is unbelievably low in calories. And fiery North African soup (page 69) is really chunky   almost more like a stew than a soup and definitely one to go for if you're used to eating hearty, meaty meals. Celeriac makes a sophisticated soup that is silky smooth and tastes amazing; try it with a trickle of truffle oil for a bit of luxury (see page 62). One thing that can make a real difference to your soup is the stock – and if you're having a go at some of the poached chicken recipes in the Chicken & Turkey chapter (pages 104–141), then you'll end up with loads of fresh, tasty home-made stock in the freezer.

Like the dressing on a salad, it's the toppings and extras that can often take a soup from a good diet option to a calorie-laden disaster. Instead of high-calorie croûtons, I've scattered chopped fresh herbs such as coriander and chives, a handful of pea shoots or some chopped spring onion or celery over the top to add a little crunch.

Try inventing your own soups by adding in whatever you have in the fridge or cupboard to the recipes in this chapter. You can work with the seasons: use root veg like carrots and turnips in winter, and summer veg like peas and courgettes in the warmer months. Lentils and beans are also great additions at any time of year, for a protein boost.

Getting organised is one of the secrets to dieting success, and most of these soups can be frozen. If you freeze them in one-person portions (use ziplock bags or plastic tubs) then you'll always have something delicious to come home to if you get in late. No more excuses for making unhealthy choices!

Salad broth

This is a really healthy, fresh-tasting lunch that won't make you feel like you need a nap in the afternoon! Lettuce and watercress may sound a bit unusual in a hot soup but just think of them as a heartier version of spinach.

Serves: 2

Calories: 235 per serving

½ tbsp olive oil
1 small red onion, sliced
3 garlic cloves, finely chopped
1 litre fresh vegetable stock
1 bouquet garni
80g new potatoes, sliced
2 medium carrots, julienned
2 little gem lettuce, shredded
50g watercress leaves (no stalks)
A handful of basil leaves,
    finely chopped
½ long red chilli, deseeded and
    finely chopped
Sea salt and freshly ground
    black pepper
2 tbsp smoked paprika dressing
    (see page 183), to finish

1. Heat the oil in a non-stick saucepan over a medium heat. Add the onion and garlic and cook for 3–4 minutes until the onion has softened.

2. Pour in the veg stock, add the bouquet garni and bring up to a simmer. Add the potatoes and carrots, and cook for 5–7 minutes or until the potatoes are soft.

3. Stir though the shredded lettuce, watercress leaves, chopped basil and red chilli. Season with salt and pepper to taste.

4. Ladle the soup into two warmed bowls. Drizzle over a little smoked paprika dressing to serve.

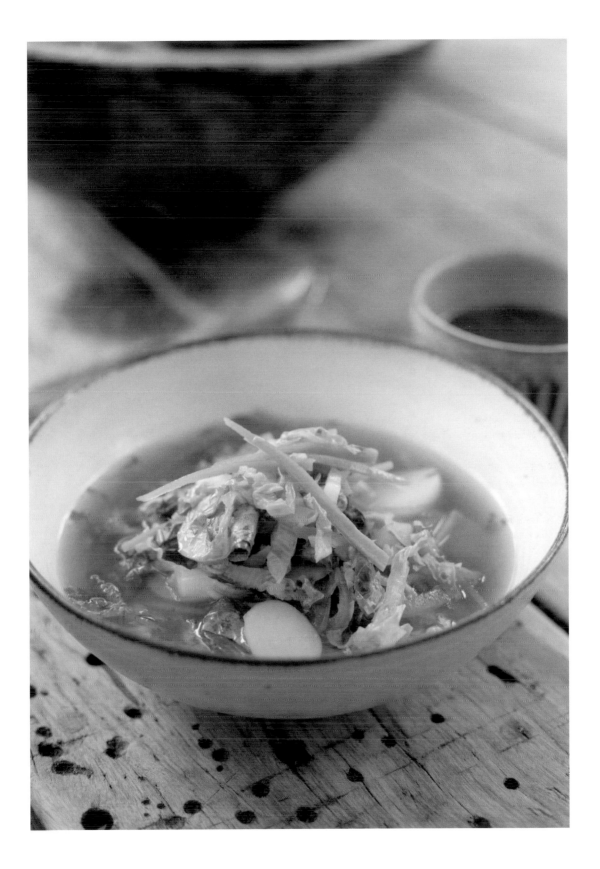

Pea and mint soup

This quick and easy soup is thickened with split peas – a good source of fibre – instead of the usual flour or potato; they also give it a fantastic richness, so you won't miss the butter. Frozen peas lend their lovely natural sweetness, balanced by fresh mint, and a final scattering of pea shoots gives an attractive finish.

Serves: 4

Calories: 315 per serving

80g yellow split peas
1 tbsp olive oil
2 large onions, finely diced
3 garlic cloves, finely chopped
2 vegetable stock cubes
1.2 litres water
700g frozen peas
2 handfuls of mint leaves,
    roughly chopped
Sea salt and freshly ground
    black pepper

To finish
4 tsp light single cream
    alternative
A handful of pea shoots

1. Put the split peas into a saucepan and pour on about 800ml water. Bring to the boil, then lower the heat and simmer for 30–45 minutes, or until just tender. Skim off any scum that rises to the surface during cooking.

2. About 10 minutes before the split peas will be cooked, heat the oil in a large saucepan over a medium heat. Add the onions and cook for 5 minutes, until softened, adding a splash of water if they start to stick. Toss in the garlic and cook for 2 minutes.

3. Drain the split peas and add them to the onions. Crumble in the veg stock cubes and pour in the 1.2 litres water. Bring to the boil, lower the heat and simmer gently for 5 minutes.

4. Now stir in the frozen peas and chopped mint. Taste the liquor, season with salt and pepper and simmer for 5 minutes, then remove from the heat.

5. Using a jug blender, blitz the soup in batches until smooth. You are aiming for a thick creamy soup. If it's a little thin, return it to the pan and simmer for a few minutes longer.

6. Ladle the soup into warmed large bowls. Drizzle over the 'cream' and finish with a scattering of fresh pea shoots.

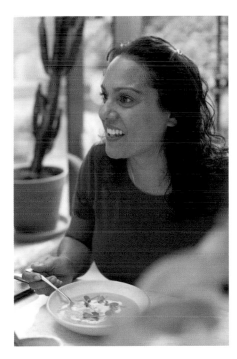

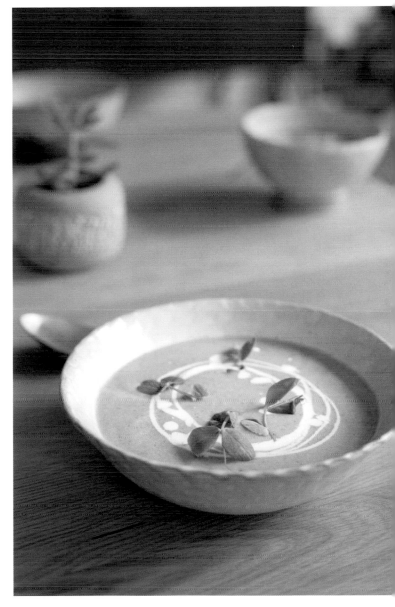

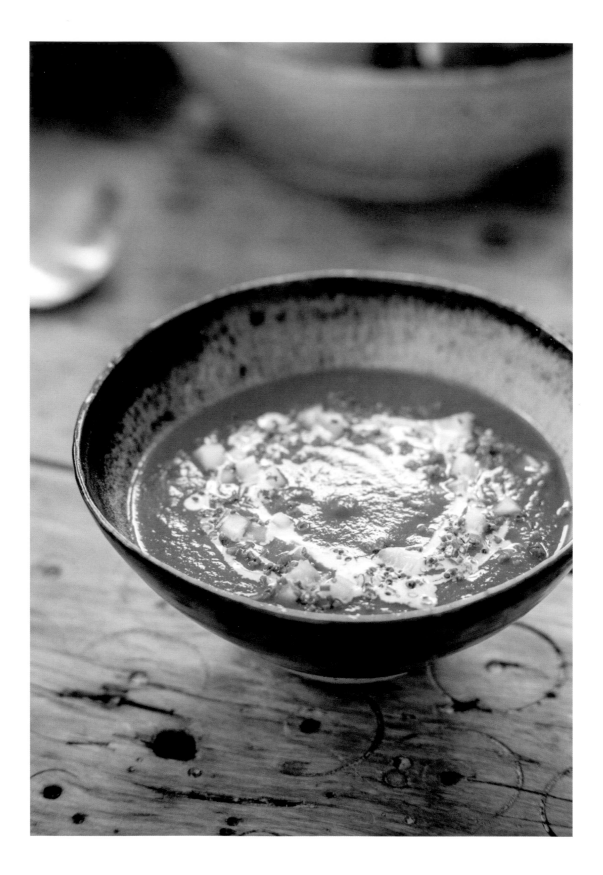

Cream of tomato soup

A creamy swirl adds a smooth, silky finish and extra richness to this soup without ramping up the calories. Get creative with your finishing touches and your soup will feel special and luxurious – here, chopped chives and celery add texture as well as another layer of flavour so you won't miss the crispy croûtons.

Serves: 4

Calories: 180 per serving

1 tbsp light olive oil
2 large onions, finely diced
6 garlic cloves, grated
2 tsp sweet smoked paprika
1 tbsp balsamic vinegar
3 x 400g tins chopped tomatoes
500ml fresh vegetable stock
1 tbsp dried herbes de Provence
1 tbsp fresh oregano, finely
   chopped
100ml light single cream
   alternative
Sea salt and freshly ground
   black pepper

To finish
1 celery stick, finely chopped
4 tbsp chopped chives
Cracked black pepper

1. Heat the oil in a large non-stick saucepan over a medium heat. Add the onions and cook for about 10 minutes until softened and golden brown. Add a splash of water if they start to stick.

2. Add the garlic and cook for 1 minute, then sprinkle in the smoked paprika and cook, stirring, for 30 seconds. Stir in the balsamic vinegar and allow it to bubble away.

3. Tip in the tinned tomatoes, pour in the veg stock and add the dried herbs and fresh oregano. Bring to the boil, then reduce the heat to a simmer and cook gently for 15 minutes – it will be quite a thick, hearty soup so loosen with a little water if you'd prefer it a little thinner.

4. Season with salt and pepper to taste and stir through half of the 'cream'. Remove from the heat. Using a jug blender, blitz the soup in batches until smooth.

5. Pour into four serving bowls and swirl the remaining 'cream' on top. Garnish with chopped celery and chives, and finish with a sprinkling of cracked black pepper.

THE LOWDOWN Most of the ingredients for this soup are ones you probably already have in your store-cupboard – so you can make it in next to no time.

Cream of celeriac soup with truffle oil

Celeriac makes a great soup as it is light but satisfying and has a lovely delicate flavour. When you're on a diet, it's really important to keep food exciting so you feel properly satisfied, stave off boredom and don't start reaching for the crisps. Here, the tiniest drizzle of truffle oil works a treat.

Serves: 4

Calories: 225 per serving

1 tbsp olive oil
3 medium onions, diced
1.2kg peeled and diced celeriac,
    (1 large or 2 small)
1.2 litres water
2 tbsp vegetable bouillon powder
4 tbsp lemon thyme leaves,
    chopped
100ml light single cream
    alternative
Sea salt and freshly ground
    black pepper

To finish
2 tsp truffle oil
Finely chopped chives

1. Heat the oil in a large non-stick saucepan over a medium heat. Add the onions and cook gently for 10 minutes or until softened but without any colour.

2. Add the celeriac, water, bouillon powder and lemon thyme. Bring to a simmer and put the lid on. Cook for about 20 minutes or until the celeriac is completely soft.

3. Using a jug blender, blitz the soup in batches until smooth. Return to the pan and place over a gentle heat. If the soup is a little thin, simmer for a few more minutes; if it's too thick, add a splash more water.

4. Taste the soup and season with salt and pepper. Stir in the 'cream' and ladle into warmed big bowls. Drizzle over the truffle oil and finish with a sprinkling of chopped chives.

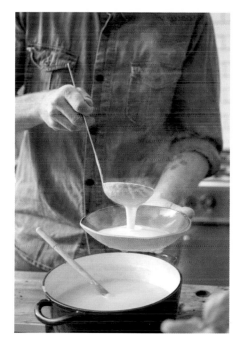

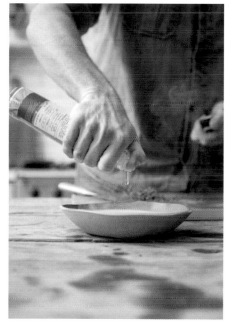

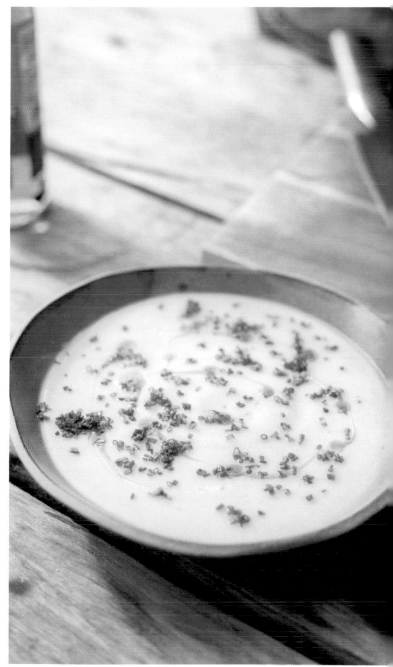

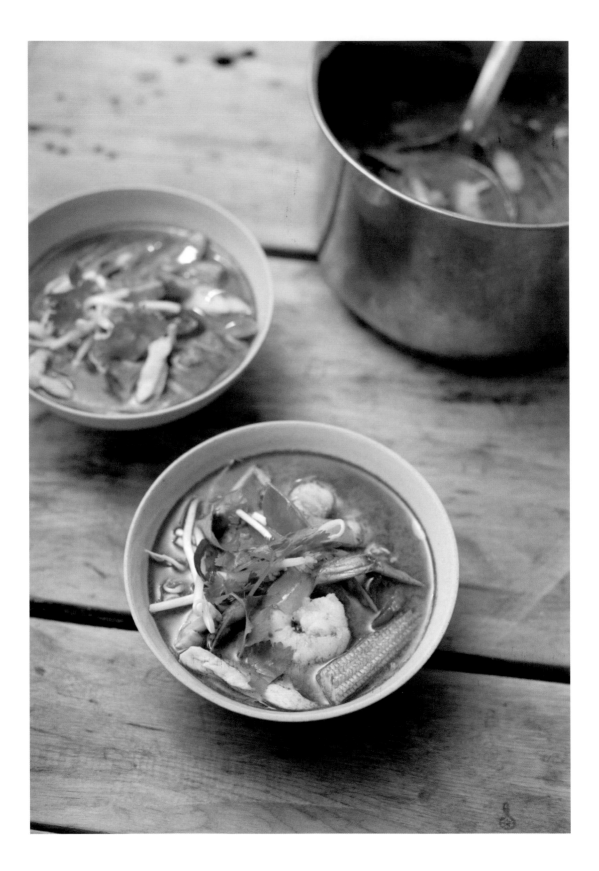

Tom yum soup

A good meal can have the power to transport you to exotic far-flung places, and this soup does exactly that. It's low in calories, yet the prawns and chicken – and ton of veggies – make it really satisfying, and it smells amazing. Like all my favourite Asian food it is perfectly balanced with just enough heat, and finished off with a refreshing squeeze of lime.

Serves: 4

Calories: 255 per serving

440g raw tiger prawns, shell on
40g galangal root, thinly sliced
2 lemongrass stems, tough outer
   layers removed and thinly sliced
4 kaffir lime leaves
1 litre fresh chicken stock
250ml water
3 tbsp good-quality tom yum paste
1 red chilli, sliced on an angle
80g button mushrooms, halved
175g baby corn, halved lengthways
200g skinless chicken breast,
   thinly sliced
80g mangetout, halved on an angle
100g bean sprouts
Juice of 1 lime
A handful of coriander leaves,
   to finish

1. Peel and devein the prawns, leaving the tails intact; cover and refrigerate. Put the prawn heads and shells into a saucepan and crush them with the end of a rolling pin to release more flavour.

2. Add the galangal, lemongrass and half the kaffir lime leaves. Pour in the chicken stock and water, bring up to a gentle simmer and simmer gently for 10 minutes.

3. Strain the stock into a clean saucepan. Stir in the tom yum paste and red chilli and bring to a simmer. Add the button mushrooms and baby corn and cook for 5 minutes, then toss in the sliced chicken and prawns and cook for 4 minutes.

4. Add the mangetout, bean sprouts and lime juice, stir through and cook for 1 minute. Check that the chicken and prawns are properly cooked, then remove from the heat.

5. Ladle the soup into warmed big bowls and scatter with coriander to serve.

Thai-style butternut squash soup

Squash is a great low-calorie veg option as it has good natural sweetness and readily takes on the flavours of other ingredients – whether that's European herbs and seasonings or, as here, some fiery, punchy spices. A really good curry paste is essential – as it forms the soup base. This is a great soup to pack into a flask and take to work.

Serves: 4

Calories: 250 per serving

1 tbsp sunflower oil
2 medium onions, diced
2 lemongrass stems, tough outer layers removed and finely sliced
3 garlic cloves, finely grated
2.5cm piece of ginger, grated
1 red chilli, finely chopped
2 tbsp good-quality Thai red curry paste (40g)
1.2kg peeled and diced butternut squash
600ml fresh vegetable stock
1 tbsp fish sauce
200ml tinned half-fat coconut milk
Sea salt and freshly ground black pepper

To finish
1 long red chilli, finely sliced
A handful of coriander leaves, roughly chopped

1. Heat the oil in a large non-stick saucepan over a high heat. Add the onions and cook for 5 minutes, adding a splash of water if they start to stick.

2. Add the lemongrass, garlic, ginger and red chilli and cook for 2 minutes, then stir in the curry paste and cook for another 1–2 minutes, until fragrant.

3. Add the butternut squash, veg stock and fish sauce and bring up to a gentle simmer. Put a lid on the pan and simmer gently for 25 minutes or until the squash has softened.

4. Pour in the coconut milk, stir well and cook, uncovered, for a further 5 minutes.

5. Using a jug blender, blitz the soup in batches until smooth. Return to the pan and place over a gentle heat. If the soup is a little thin, simmer for a few minutes more; if it's too thick, add a splash more water.

6. Taste the soup and season with salt and pepper if needed. Divide between warmed bowls and top with sliced red chilli and chopped coriander. Grind a little extra black pepper over each serving too.

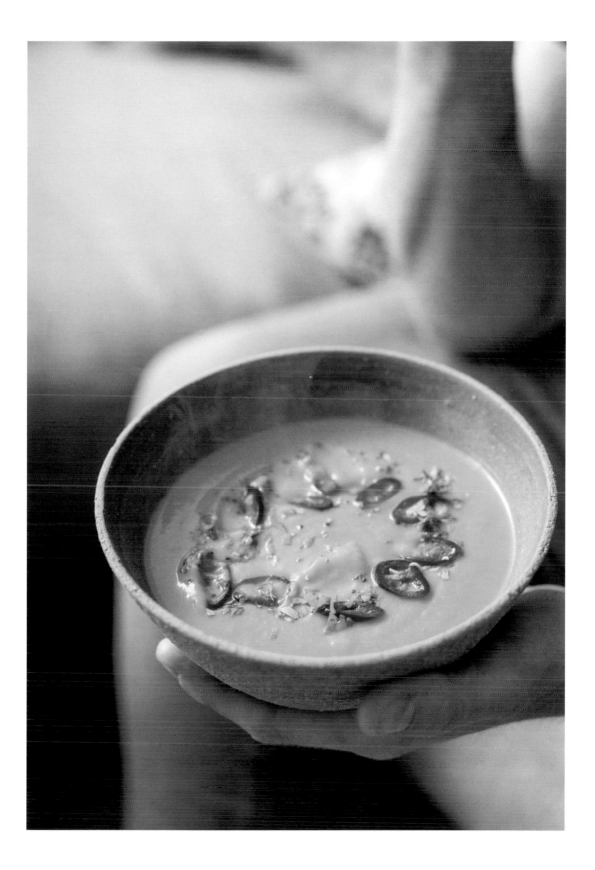

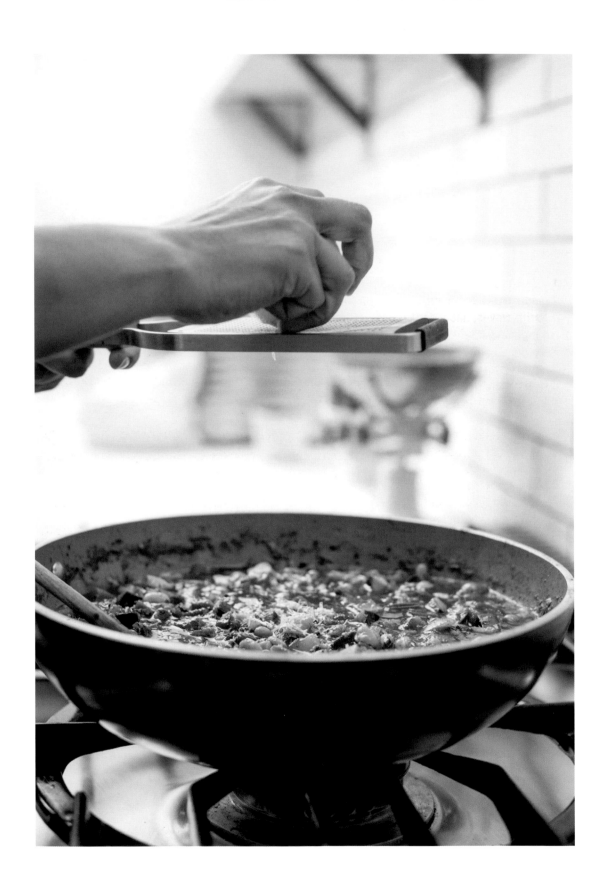

North African soup

Think of this soup like a minestrone but with lots of big, bold North African flavours. Rose harissa is a fantastic ingredient to keep in your fridge – the smallest amount brings so many extra layers of taste. Chickpeas and aubergine add body, replacing the need for pasta or meat to make this a satisfying one-bowl meal.

Serves: 4

Calories: 235 per serving

1 tbsp olive oil
2 medium onions, diced
4 garlic cloves, finely chopped
2 tsp ground cumin
1 tsp ground coriander
3 tsp rose harissa paste
2 tbsp tomato purée
1.2 litres fresh vegetable stock
400g tin chopped tomatoes
450g aubergines, diced
300g courgettes, diced
400g tin chickpeas, rinsed and
   drained (240g drained weight)
150g frozen broad beans
2 handfuls of coriander leaves,
   roughly chopped
Finely grated zest of 1 lemon
Sea salt and freshly ground
   black pepper

1. Heat the oil in a large non-stick saucepan over a high heat. When hot, add the onions and cook for 5 minutes, adding a splash of water if they start to stick. Add the garlic and cook for 2 minutes, stirring occasionally.

2. Lower the heat a little and stir through the cumin and ground coriander. Cook, stirring, for 1 minute and then add the rose harissa and tomato purée and stir over the heat for another minute.

3. Add the veg stock, tinned tomatoes, aubergines, courgettes and chickpeas. Bring to the boil, lower the heat and simmer for 20–30 minutes.

4. Add the broad beans, chopped coriander and lemon zest. Remove from the heat and season with salt and pepper to taste. Ladle into warmed large bowls to serve.

THE LOWDOWN Like frozen peas, frozen broad beans taste fresh all year round as they are frozen quickly after picking. Keep a bag in your freezer to add extra texture and taste to stews, soups and casseroles.

Chicken and sweetcorn soup

The ever-popular classic Chinese soup is based on just two main ingredients – chicken and sweetcorn. This recipe extracts as much flavour out of each one as possible, using the corn cooking water as part of the stock for the soup. It is thickened with cornflour and has egg swirled through for extra taste and texture.

Serves: 4

Calories: 385 per serving

4 corn-on-the-cob (about 200g each)
1 skinless chicken crown (750g), pre-poached in 500ml fresh chicken stock and 500ml water then cooled (see page 105)
½ tbsp vegetable oil
½ tbsp sesame oil
2 medium onions, finely chopped
2 garlic cloves, finely chopped
5cm piece of ginger, finely grated
500ml fresh chicken stock (reserved from poaching the chicken)
2 tbsp cornflour, mixed to a paste with 2 tbsp water
1 tbsp light soy sauce
¼ tsp freshly ground white pepper
1 large free-range egg, lightly beaten
4 spring onions, finely sliced on an angle
Flaky sea salt

1. Place the corn-on-the-cob in a large saucepan and cover with at least 1 litre water. Bring to the boil, lower the heat and simmer for 20–25 minutes or until the corn is cooked. Leave the cobs to cool in the water.

2. Once cooled, remove the corn cobs, reserving 500ml water of the liquor (i.e. flavourful corn stock). Carefully run a knife down the corn cobs to remove all the juicy corn kernels. Set them aside.

3. Take the chicken breasts off the bone and tear the meat into shreds.

4. Place a large non-stick saucepan over a high heat. When hot, add the oils, then the chopped onions and sauté for 5 minutes, adding a splash of water if they start to stick. Add the garlic and ginger and cook for 2 minutes.

5. Pour in the chicken stock and reserved corn stock and bring up to a simmer. Add the shredded chicken and sweetcorn kernels and bring back to a simmer. Stir in the cornflour paste and cook, stirring, for a minute or two, until the soup thickens slightly. Season with the soy sauce, white pepper and a little flaky salt.

6. Pour in the beaten egg, stirring well to create thin strands. Add half of the spring onions. Ladle the soup into warmed bowls and scatter over the remaining spring onions to serve.

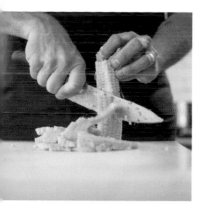

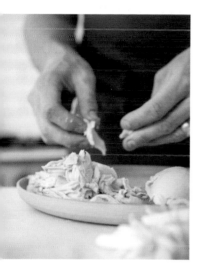

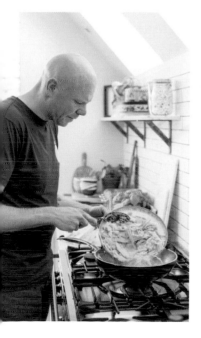

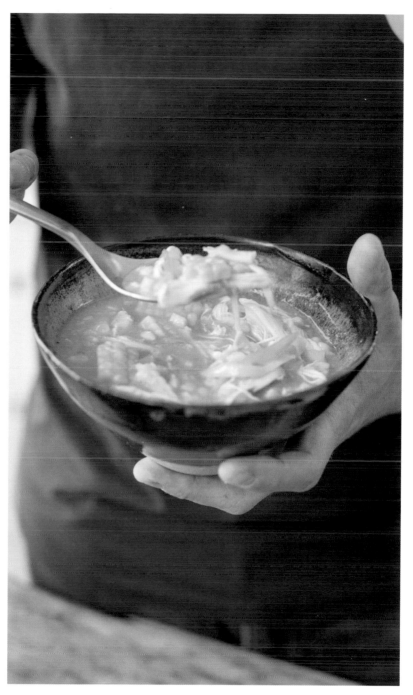

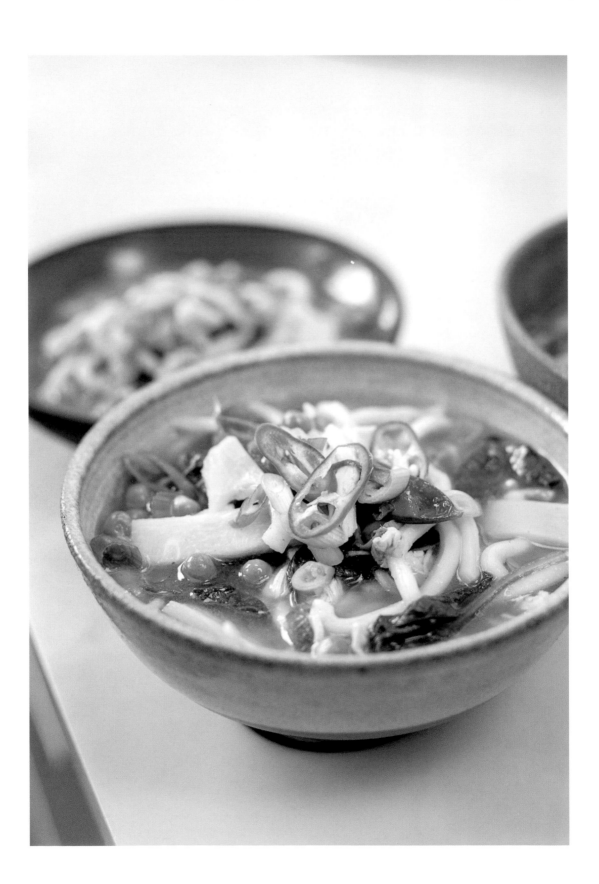

Asian chicken and pea broth

This warming, fragrant broth is packed with flavour from the lemongrass, lime leaves, ginger, curry paste and coconut milk. There's a lot going on here with the texture too – crunchy veg, meaty chicken and the noodles make it so satisfying to eat. It's about as far from regular diet food as you can get!

Serves: 4

Calories: 490 per serving

1 skinless chicken crown (750g), pre-poached in 500ml fresh chicken stock and 500ml water then cooled (see page 105)
400g fresh peas in their pods, rinsed
1.5 litres fresh chicken stock (include the stock reserved from poaching the chicken)
6 garlic cloves, grated
2.5cm piece of ginger, finely grated
2 lemongrass stems, lightly bashed
4 kaffir lime leaves
2 tbsp good-quality Thai green curry paste (40g)
150ml tinned half-fat coconut milk
1 tbsp fish sauce
100g mangetout
225g tin bamboo shoots, drained
300g straight-to-wok udon noodles
200g bean sprouts
150g baby spinach
6 spring onions, finely sliced on an angle
1 green chilli, finely sliced on an angle, to finish

1. Take the chicken breasts off the bone and tear the meat into shreds; set aside.

2. Pod the peas and place all the pods in a large saucepan; set the peas aside for later. Pour the chicken stock over the pea pods and add the garlic, ginger, lemongrass and lime leaves. Bring to a low simmer and cook gently for 10 minutes.

3. Strain the stock and then return it to the large saucepan. Bring to a gentle simmer and stir in the curry paste, coconut milk and fish sauce. Toss in the chicken, mangetout, bamboo shoots and udon noodles and cook for 4–5 minutes.

4. Meanwhile, put a small handful of bean sprouts into the bottom of each serving bowl.

5. Stir the spinach, peas and spring onions through the soup, then ladle over the bean sprouts in the bowls. Top with sliced green chilli and serve.

Veg and lentil soup

Red lentils can be cooked out to a soft, creamy soup that is really sustaining – perfect for dieting in winter. The classic combination of onion, carrot and celery provides the soup base, with lentils rather than potatoes thickening the stock. It's also a great soup to keep in the freezer for a quick substantial meal to stop you reaching for a takeaway if you're home late.

Serves: 4

Calories: 450 per serving

1 tbsp olive oil
4 medium onions, diced
4 medium carrots, diced
5 celery sticks, diced
10 garlic cloves, finely chopped
3 tbsp thyme leaves, chopped
350g red lentils, well washed
   and drained
45g vegetable bouillon powder
1.8 litres water
Sea salt and freshly ground
   black pepper

1. Heat the oil in a large non-stick saucepan over a high heat. Add the onions and sauté for 5 minutes, adding a splash of water if they start to stick. Add the carrots and cook for 2 minutes, then toss in the celery and garlic and cook for another 2 minutes, stirring occasionally.

2. Add the thyme, lentils, bouillon powder and water. Season with plenty of pepper. Stir and bring to the boil, then lower the heat to a simmer. Cook, stirring occasionally, for 15 minutes or until the lentils have softened, skimming off any scum that rises to the surface.

3. Ladle half of the soup into a jug blender and blitz until smooth. Return the blended soup to the pan and stir well.

4. Taste to check the seasoning and adjust if necessary, then ladle the soup into warmed big bowls. Grind over a little extra pepper to serve.

....

THE LOWDOWN Lentils are a great, cheap source of low-calorie protein, especially if you're cutting down on meat. They take on flavours really well too – so keep a bag in your cupboard to bulk out stews and soups.

....

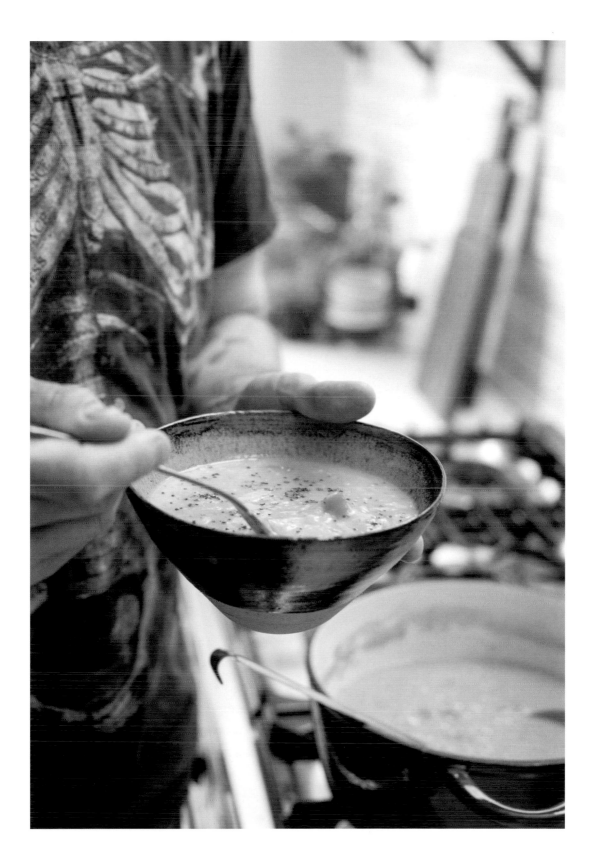

FISH & SEAFOOD

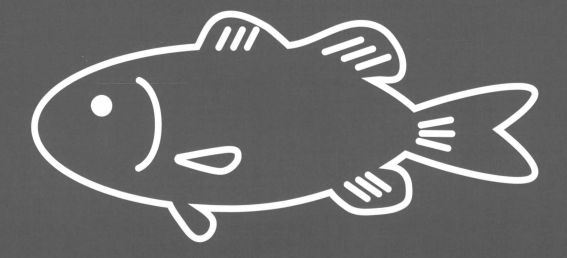

Fish and seafood are healthy foods but most of us don't eat enough of them. High in protein, yet low in calories and fat, while fish and prawns are great choices when you're on a diet. Oily fish, like salmon and tuna, are good for you too, as they are a rich source of those all-important omega-3s – just be aware that they are higher in calories than white fish. That said, they taste so rich, you won't need much to feel you've eaten something substantial.

The trick with fish is to prevent it from drying out as it cooks, so it keeps lovely and moist. It's easy to do this, without introducing buttery or creamy sauces. One-pot stews, curries and traybakes are all great ways to keep fish succulent. There are lots of them in this chapter, such as Thai red prawn curry (page 85), Baked cod with beans, courgettes and chorizo (page 93) and Italian seafood pot (page 94). Cooking everything together not only helps the fish to stay moist, it also makes the finished dish taste extra delicious because all the fantastic flavours mingle together.

Another clever way of keeping in the moisture is to cook your fish in a paper parcel – try my easy Fish-in-a-bag Chinese-style (page 88), which is ready on the table in under half an hour.

If you're buying fresh fish, try to get the best quality you can, as it makes all the difference to the finished dish. Get to know your fishmonger and they can let you know when the next delivery is on its way.

It's preferable to use fresh fish, of course, but if you stash a bag of frozen prawns in the freezer then you know you can have a tasty meal ready to go in minutes. If you keep a bag of frozen peas in there too you're halfway to making my Prawn curry with peas (page 78). And having a tin of good-quality tuna in the cupboard means you've got the base for the chunky fish cakes on page 97 at the ready too.

Keeping mealtimes varied and exciting is the secret to dieting success, and the beauty of fish and seafood is that they work with lots of different flavours – whether that's zingy hints of lemon or lime, heady Asian or Indian spices or the sun-drenched taste of Mediterranean herbs. Whatever you go for, your Friday night fish supper just got a whole lot more interesting!

Prawn curry with peas

Prawns are a great low-calorie ingredient – they are quick to prepare with a distinct flavour of their own and a satisfying meaty texture. You can even use frozen prawns here, defrosting them fully first. Adding a pinch of saffron to the rice as it cooks not only results in an amazing golden colour but adds an extra layer of taste – I always look for ways of getting more flavour into food whenever I can.

Serves: 2

Calories: 345 per serving

½ tbsp vegetable oil
1 tsp black mustard seeds
1 tsp cumin seeds
1 large onion, finely diced
1 green chilli, finely chopped
2 garlic cloves, finely grated
2.5cm piece of ginger, finely grated
A handful of curry leaves
    (ideally fresh, but dried will do)
200g tomatoes, finely diced
A large pinch of saffron strands
300ml fresh fish stock
150ml tinned half-fat coconut milk
350g raw tiger prawns, peeled and
    deveined, leaving the tail on
100g frozen peas
100g baby spinach
Sea salt and freshly ground
    black pepper

To serve
160g basmati rice, cooked
    with salt and a pinch of
    saffron strands

1. Heat the oil in a medium non-stick sauté pan or wok over a high heat. When hot, add the mustard and cumin seeds. When they begin to pop, add the onion and sauté until just starting to brown. Toss in the green chilli, garlic, ginger and curry leaves and cook for 2 minutes.

2. Stir in the tomatoes and saffron and cook for 2–3 minutes or until the tomatoes have softened.

3. Pour in the fish stock and let it bubble until reduced by half, then add the coconut milk and cook for 5 minutes.

4. Add the prawns and peas, and cook until the prawns begin to turn pink. Stir in the spinach and season with salt and pepper to taste, then check that the prawns are cooked.

5. Divide the curry between warmed bowls and serve with the saffron rice on the side.

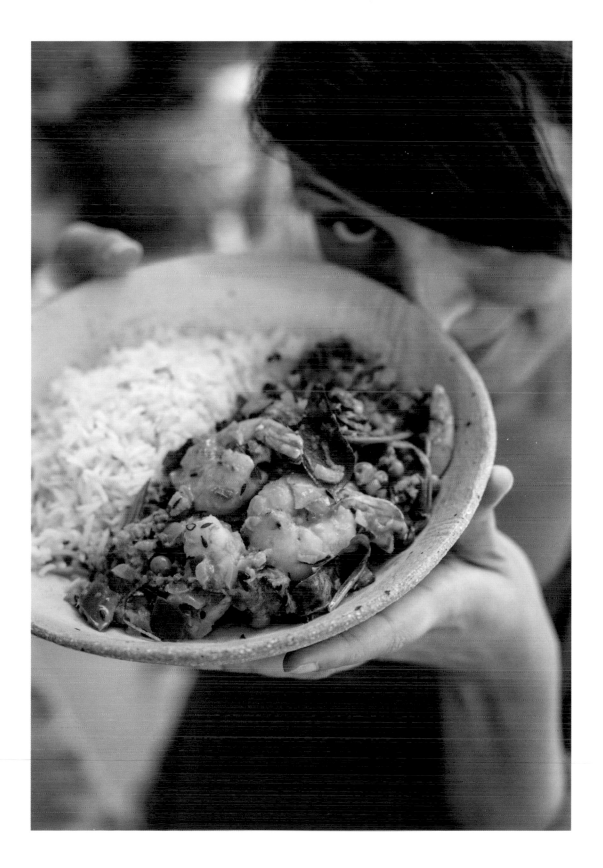

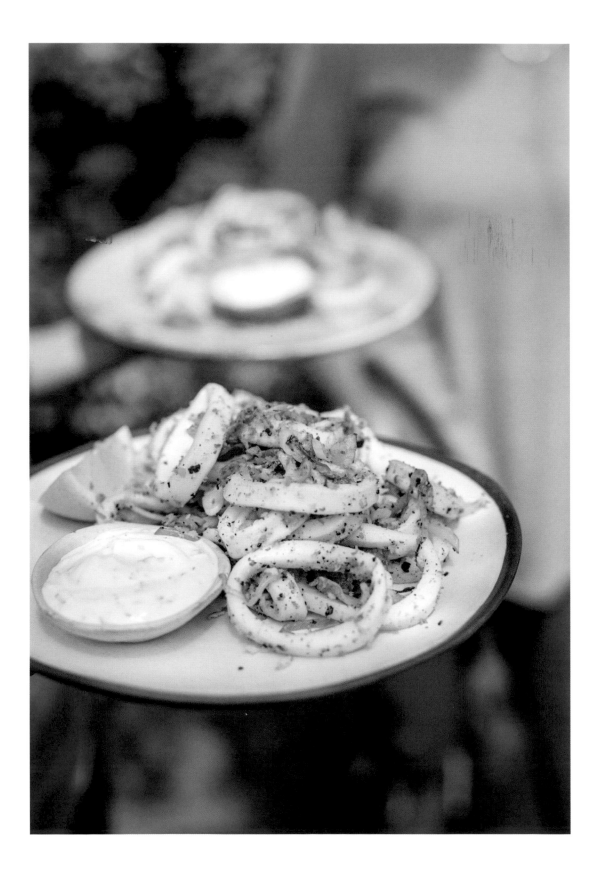

Salt and pepper squid with yuzu mayo

This is a great way of cooking squid to achieve that satisfying crunchy texture, but without coating it in breadcrumbs and deep-frying. Yuzu is a Japanese citrus fruit with a wonderful intense taste – you need only a little of the juice to give the fresh, lower fat dip a fantastic flavour.

Serves: 2

Calories: 275 per serving

1 tsp Szechuan peppercorns
½ tsp black peppercorns
1 tsp flaky sea salt
½ tbsp light olive oil
½ onion, thinly sliced
1 garlic clove, thinly sliced
30g panko dried breadcrumbs
1 red chilli, finely sliced
2 spring onions, finely sliced
   on an angle
350g squid rings

For the yuzu mayo
1 tsp yuzu juice
1½ tbsp half-fat mayonnaise
3 tbsp Greek yoghurt (0% fat)
1 tbsp finely chopped coriander

To serve
Lemon or lime wedges

1. Coarsely grind all the peppercorns together, using a pestle and mortar. Tip into a small bowl, stir in the salt and set aside.

2. For the yuzu mayo, put all the ingredients into a small bowl, stir to combine and set aside.

3. Heat a non-stick wok over a high heat. When hot, add the oil, then the onion and garlic. Cook for about 5 minutes, until the onion is softened. Add the breadcrumbs and chilli and stir-fry until the crumbs turn golden brown. Remove from the heat and stir through the spring onions. Tip out onto a plate and set aside.

4. Place the wok back over a very high heat and give it a couple of minutes to heat up. When it is very hot, add the squid rings and stir them around quickly until they release their liquid. This will only take a couple of minutes.

5. Sprinkle the salt and pepper mix over the squid – depending on how spicy you like it, you may not need all of it. Stir in the breadcrumb mix, then take the pan off the heat.

6. Serve the squid straight away, with the yuzu mayonnaise alongside and lemon or lime wedges for squeezing.

South Indian fish curry

This is a light dish but it is overflowing with layer upon layer of aromatics. You can replace the cod with haddock or hake if you like.

Serves: 4

Calories: 425 per serving

800g skinless cod fillets
1 tbsp table salt
1 tbsp vegetable oil
2 tsp black mustard seeds
1 tsp cumin seeds
2 onions, finely diced
A handful of curry leaves
    (ideally fresh, but dried will do)
4 garlic cloves, finely chopped
4cm piece of ginger, finely grated
2 long green chillies, finely
    chopped
1 tsp ground turmeric
1 tsp ground coriander
4 large tomatoes, diced
500ml fresh fish stock
200ml tinned full-fat coconut milk
200g tenderstem broccoli, stalks
    cut in half
250g frozen peas
Sea salt and freshly ground
    black pepper

To finish (optional)
½ lime, to spritz
Coriander leaves, roughly chopped

1. Sprinkle the cod fillets on both sides with the table salt and leave for 20 minutes.

2. Heat the oil in a large non-stick sauté pan over a high heat then add the mustard and cumin seeds. When they begin to pop and crackle, add the diced onions and cook for 5 minutes or until softened and starting to brown. Toss in the curry leaves, garlic, ginger and chillies and stir-fry for 1–2 minutes. Add a splash of water if the mixture starts to stick.

3. Lower the heat and add the ground spices with a little salt and pepper. Cook, stirring, for 1 minute then add the tomatoes and cook for 2–3 minutes until they start to break down. Pour in the stock and simmer for about 20 minutes, until reduced by half.

4. Wash the salt off the fish, pat dry with kitchen paper and cut into 5–6cm pieces.

5. Stir the coconut milk into the curry mixture and continue to simmer for 5–10 minutes until reduced by one-third. Add the fish and broccoli and simmer gently for about 5 minutes, until just cooked.

6. Stir through the peas and taste to check the seasoning. Serve in warmed large bowls, adding a squeeze of lime and a scattering of coriander if you like.

....

THE LOWDOWN Salting fish before cooking firms it up, resulting in a meatier and more satisfying texture.

....

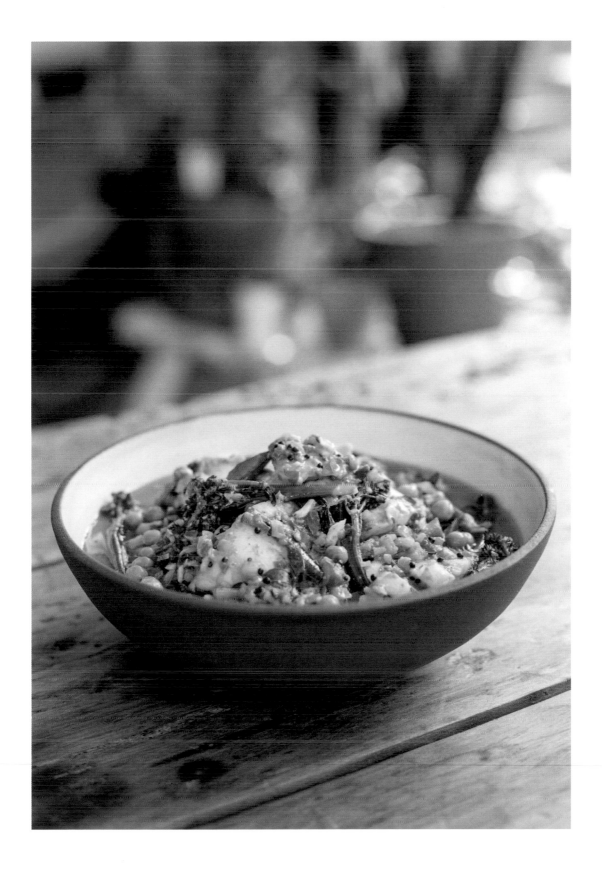

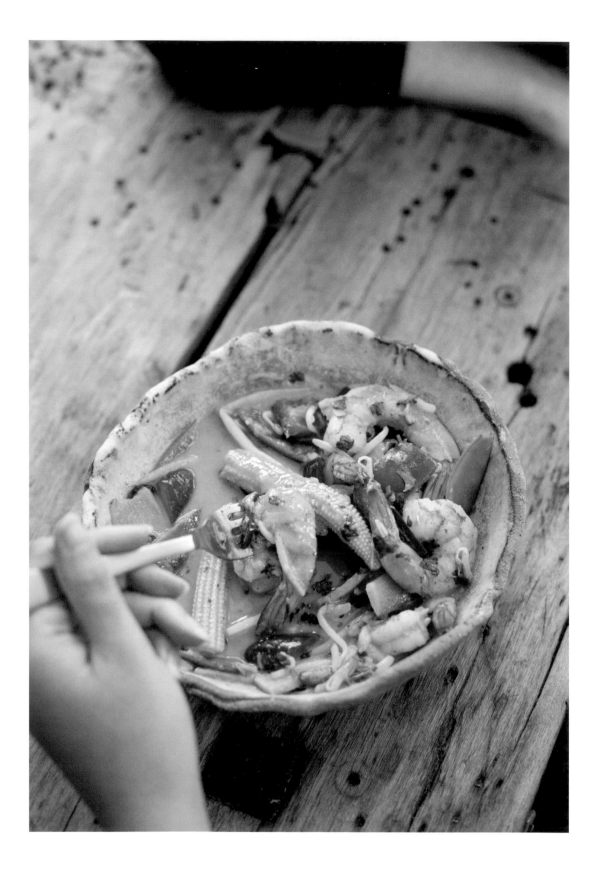

Thai red prawn curry

Don't underestimate how important your sense of smell is to your enjoyment of food – this fragrant curry is a treat for *all* the senses! With so much going on, thanks to the big authentic flavours, creamy coconut milk and crunchy veg, you won't miss having rice on the side.

Serves: 4

Calories: 400 per serving

750g raw tiger prawns, shell on
500ml fresh fish stock
250ml water
1 lemongrass stem, bashed and halved lengthways
4 kaffir lime leaves
1 tbsp vegetable oil
1 large onion, sliced
4 garlic cloves, finely chopped
2.5cm piece of ginger, finely grated
3 tbsp good-quality Thai red curry paste (60g)
300ml tinned full-fat coconut milk
175g baby corn, halved lengthways
1 large red pepper, cored, deseeded and cut into large dice
100g mangetout or sugar snap peas, halved
120g drained tinned bamboo shoots
100g bean sprouts
A handful of coriander, roughly chopped
1 long red chilli, finely sliced (optional)

1. Peel and devein the prawns, leaving the tails intact; set aside. Place the heads and shells in a saucepan and pour on the fish stock and water to cover. Add the lemongrass and 2 kaffir lime leaves. Bring to the boil and simmer until the liquor has reduced by half.

2. Heat the oil in a large non-stick wok. Add the onion and stir-fry for 2–3 minutes, then toss in the garlic and ginger and stir-fry for another 2 minutes. Stir in the curry paste and cook for 1 minute, stirring all the time.

3. Strain the prawn stock through a fine sieve, discarding the shells, and pour into the wok. Add the remaining kaffir lime leaves and bring to the boil. Pour in the coconut milk, add the baby corn and simmer for 5 minutes.

4. Add the red pepper, mangetout, bamboo shoots and prawns. Bring to a simmer and simmer gently for 5 minutes or until the prawns are cooked.

5. Remove the pan from the heat and stir in the bean sprouts and coriander. Serve in warmed large bowls, sprinkled with sliced red chilli for an extra bit of heat if you like.

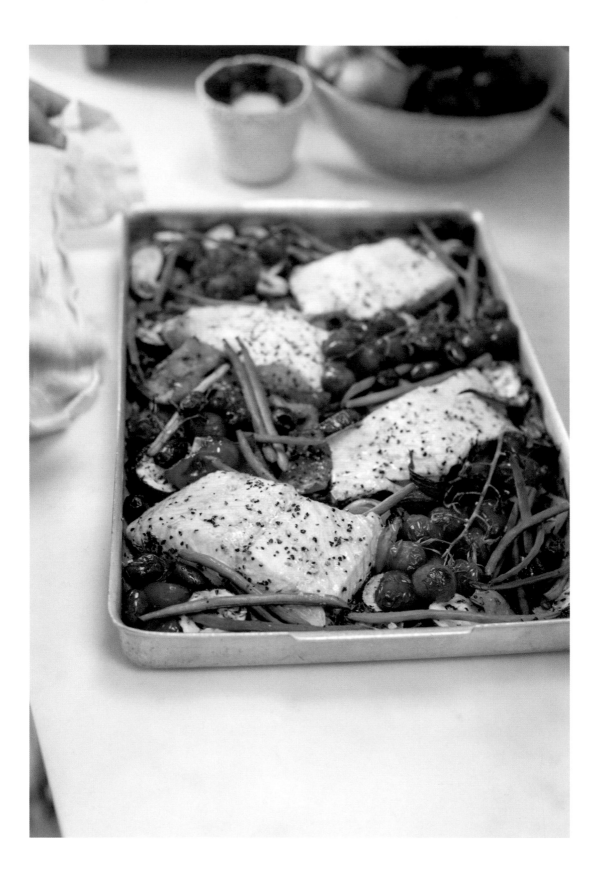

Provençal salmon traybake

Traybakes are such a time-saver when you're on a diet. Just whack it all in the oven and let it do its thing – no need to stress about it! The only thing to be a bit careful of is not to overcook the salmon.

Serves: 4

Calories: 560 per serving

1 large red onion, cut into
    12 wedges
12 garlic cloves, peeled but
    left whole
1 large red pepper, cored,
    deseeded and cut into
    3cm chunks
1 large yellow pepper, cored,
    deseeded and cut into
    3cm chunks
2 large courgettes, cut into
    1cm slices
1 tsp dried herbes de Provence
2 tbsp fresh oregano, finely
    chopped
Olive oil spray
120g fine green beans
4 skinless salmon fillets
    (200g each)
200g cherry tomatoes on the vine
50g pitted black olives
100ml fresh fish stock
Sea salt and freshly ground
    black pepper
A handful of basil leaves, to finish
    (optional)

1. Preheat the oven to fan 220°C/gas 7.

2. Scatter the onion, garlic, peppers, courgettes, dried herbs and fresh oregano in a roasting tray. Season generously with salt and pepper and spray 25 times with oil. Mix well and cook on the top shelf of the oven for 20 minutes.

3. Meanwhile, add the green beans to a small pan of boiling salted water and blanch for a couple of minutes until cooked but still firm to the bite. Drain and immerse in a bowl of cold water to cool quickly, then drain well.

4. Remove the tray from oven and nestle the salmon fillets, cherry tomatoes, green beans and olives in amongst the roasted vegetables. Pour over the fish stock. Sprinkle the salmon with salt and pepper and spray with another 20 sprays of oil.

5. Return the roasting tray to the top shelf of the oven and bake for about 10–15 minutes, until the salmon is cooked. Serve, scattered with basil leaves if you like.

Fish-in-a-bag Chinese style

Cooking *'en papillote'* like this seals in flavour and moisture and is a great way to make white fish taste more exciting without using batter, breadcrumbs or a buttery sauce. A quick and easy technique, it has the added bonus of less washing up!

Serves: 4

Calories: 550 per serving

6 tbsp light soy sauce
3 tbsp Shaoxing wine
24 Szechuan peppercorns,
    lightly crushed
3 tbsp water
1 tbsp cornflour, mixed to a paste
    with 1 tbsp water
4 baby pak choi, halved
    lengthways
8 tenderstem broccoli stalks
2 handfuls of bean sprouts (140g)
4 sea bass fillets (150g each)
4 large garlic cloves, thinly sliced
12cm piece of ginger, julienned
1 red chilli, sliced on an angle
Sea salt and freshly ground
    white pepper

To serve
240g jasmine rice, cooked

1. Preheat the oven to fan 200°C/gas 6. Cut four pieces of baking parchment, about 40 x 35cm.

2. Put the soy sauce, Shaoxing wine, Szechuan peppercorns and the 3 tbsp water into a small pan and bring to a simmer over a medium heat. Remove from the heat and whisk in the cornflour paste, then return to the heat and whisk until the mixture has thickened to the consistency of ketchup. Set aside.

3. Lay one halved pak choi in the middle of each piece of baking parchment and top with the broccoli and bean sprouts. Season the fish with salt and white pepper and place a fillet on each pile of veg.

4. Scatter the garlic, ginger and red chilli on top of the fish, then spoon over the sauce. Bring the long edges of the paper together over the fish and fold them together to seal, scrunching the ends to close these too. Place on a baking tray and cook in the oven for 18–20 minutes.

5. Lift each bag onto a warmed serving plate, to rip open at the table. Serve with jasmine rice.

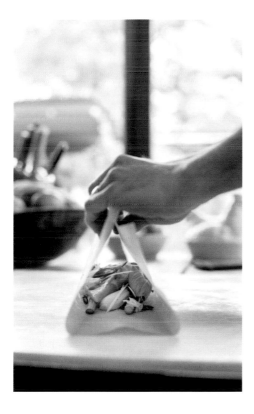

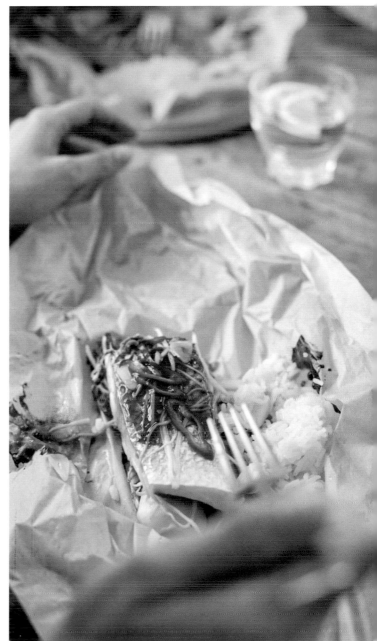

THE LOWDOWN Sea bass is great here, but you could use any fish you like: hake, cod, haddock or even salmon. Just be aware that whatever you use will affect the calorie count.

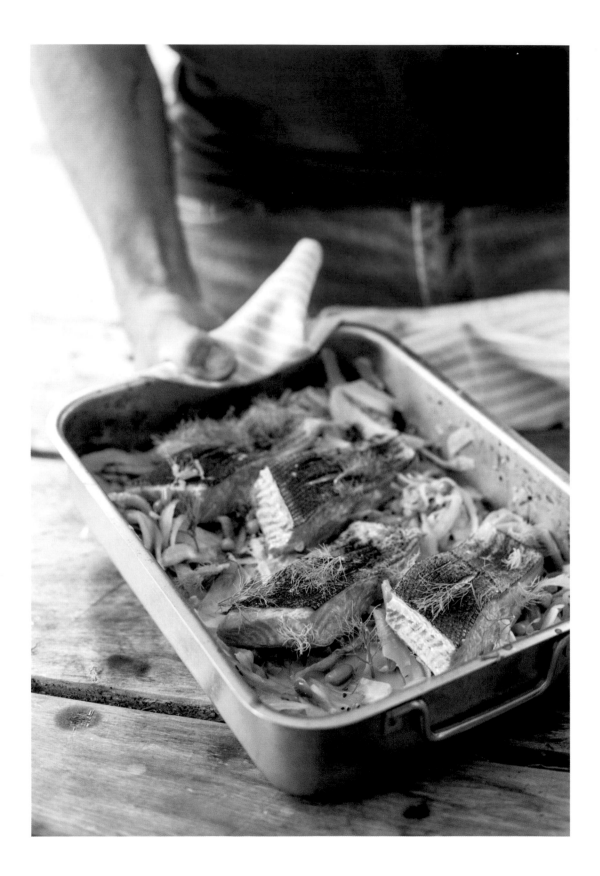

Rainbow trout with braised fennel

Rainbow trout is a brilliant British fish that is sadly underused. It has a delicate flavour that pairs well with fennel, peas and broad beans in this traybake. Just make sure the fish is very fresh. If you can't get hold of rainbow trout, you can use salmon instead, although the calories will be a bit higher.

Serves: 2

Calories: 500 per serving

2 medium fennel bulbs, thinly
    sliced, fronds reserved
2 banana shallots, thinly sliced
3 garlic cloves, finely sliced
250ml fresh fish stock
4 skin-on rainbow trout fillets
    (120g each)
100g frozen peas
100g frozen baby broad beans
Finely grated zest of 1 lemon
2 tbsp crème fraîche
Sea salt and freshly ground
    black pepper

1. Preheat the oven to fan 180°C/gas 4.

2. Put the fennel, shallots and garlic into a roasting tin, mix well and season with salt and pepper. Pour on the fish stock and cover the tin with foil. Cook on the top shelf of the oven for 15 minutes, taking out the roasting tin halfway through to give everything a good stir and stop the fennel burning.

3. Remove the foil and return the roasting tin to the oven for 10 minutes until the fennel is cooked and there is only a little liquid left. If necessary, give it a few more minutes in the oven.

4. Meanwhile, season both sides of the trout with salt and pepper then, with a sharp knife, score the skin at 1cm intervals. Place the fish, skin side up, on a metal tray and wave a cook's blowtorch over the skin until lightly charred.

5. Remove the roasting tin from the oven and add the peas, broad beans and lemon zest. Lay the trout on top of the fennel and bake for 5 minutes or until the trout is just cooked through.

6. Mix the crème fraîche through the fennel and scatter the reserved fennel fronds over the trout. Serve straight away.

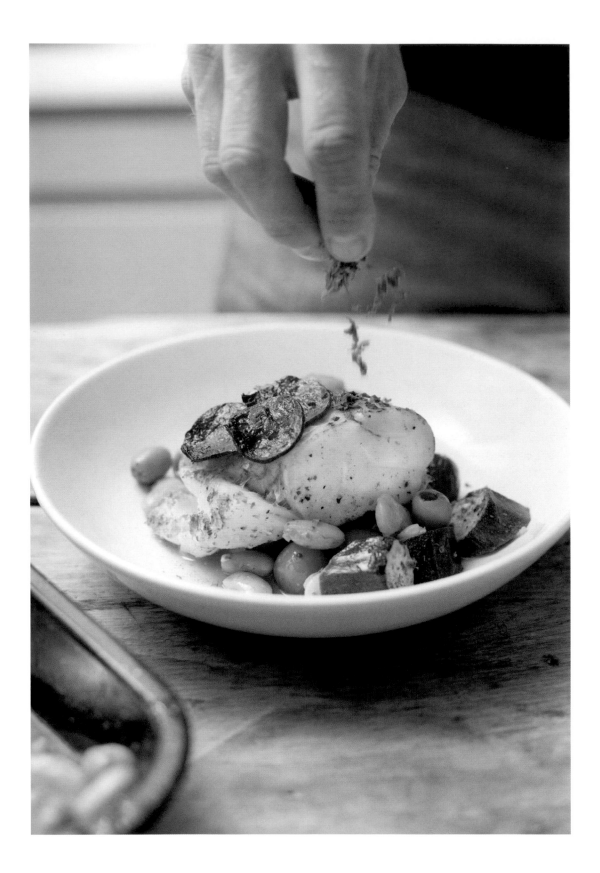

Baked cod with beans, courgettes and chorizo

Feeling that you are depriving yourself on a diet is a short trip down the road to giving up entirely. Don't do it to yourself! Although there's not much chorizo in this dish, it gives such a tasty, crispy extra layer that you won't feel you're missing out.

Serves: 2

Calories: 535 per serving

2 tsp flaky sea salt
1 tsp hot smoked paprika
2 cod fillets (200g each)
3 medium courgettes, cut
   into chunks
4 garlic cloves, thickly sliced
200ml fresh fish stock
1 tsp dried oregano
Olive oil spray
400g tin butter beans, rinsed
   and drained
200g cherry tomatoes on the vine
40g pitted green olives
8 thin slices of chorizo
Finely grated zest and juice of
   1 lemon
Sea salt and freshly ground
   black pepper
Flat-leaf parsley, finely chopped,
   to finish

1. Mix the flaky salt with ½ tsp smoked paprika and sprinkle over both sides of the cod fillets. Place them on a plate, cover with cling film and refrigerate for 1–2 hours.

2. Preheat the oven to fan 180°C/gas 4. Line a roasting tin with baking parchment.

3. Place the courgettes in the roasting tin. Add the garlic and pour on half of the fish stock. Sprinkle with the oregano and some salt and pepper. Spray with 25–30 sprays of oil. Cook on the middle shelf of the oven for 15 minutes.

4. Remove the fish from the fridge, wash off the salt and pat dry with kitchen paper.

5. Take the tray from the oven and mix through the butter beans. Nestle the fish fillets into the mixture, along with the cherry tomatoes and olives. Pour on the rest of the fish stock. Lay the chorizo slices, overlapping, on top of the cod fillets.

6. Sprinkle the lemon zest and juice and the remaining ½ tsp smoked paprika over everything and season with salt and pepper. Spray another 20 sprays of oil over the surface and bake in the oven for 12 minutes, until the fish is just cooked. Sprinkle with chopped parsley and serve.

Italian seafood pot

This relatively quick one-pot wonder locks in all the flavours of the Med, packing in the taste of great summer holidays! The trick is to cut all the veggies about the same size so they cook evenly, but be careful not to overcook them – you want them to retain some bite. Smoked cod adds another layer of amazing flavour.

Serves: 4

Calories: 400 per serving

1 tbsp mild olive oil
2 medium onions, finely diced
2 medium fennel bulbs, finely diced, fronds reserved
4 garlic cloves, finely chopped
1 tsp fennel seeds
½ tsp dried chilli flakes
A big pinch of saffron strands
500ml fresh fish stock
2 x 400g tins chopped tomatoes
2 large courgettes, finely diced
80g pitted kalamata olives, halved
1½ tbsp baby capers
100g orzo pasta
400g smoked cod fillet, cut into 2cm slices
250g raw tiger prawns, peeled and deveined, leaving the tail on
Sea salt and freshly ground black pepper

1. Heat the oil in a large non-stick frying pan over a medium-high heat. Add the onions and cook for 5–7 minutes or until softened, adding a splash of water if they start to stick.

2. Toss in the diced fennel and garlic and cook for 4–5 minutes or until starting to brown. Add the fennel seeds, chilli flakes and saffron, stir well and cook for 1 minute.

3. Pour in the fish stock, tip in the tinned tomatoes and bring to the boil. Add the courgettes, olives, capers and orzo, stir well and reduce to a gentle simmer. Cook for 10–12 minutes or until the pasta is nearly cooked.

4. Add the smoked cod slices, tiger prawns and some salt and pepper. Stir well and cook for about 5 minutes, until the seafood is just cooked. Taste to check the seasoning and serve in warmed bowls, sprinkled with the reserved fennel fronds.

•••

THE LOWDOWN Cutting the veg as small as possible gives it the texture of rice or orzo – you will think you are eating more orzo but it's far fewer calories!

•••

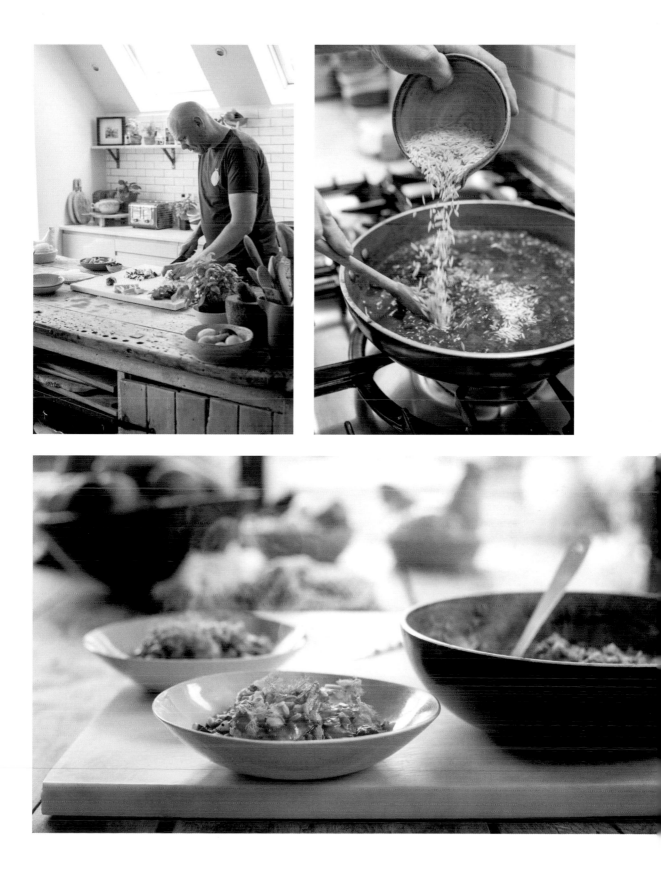

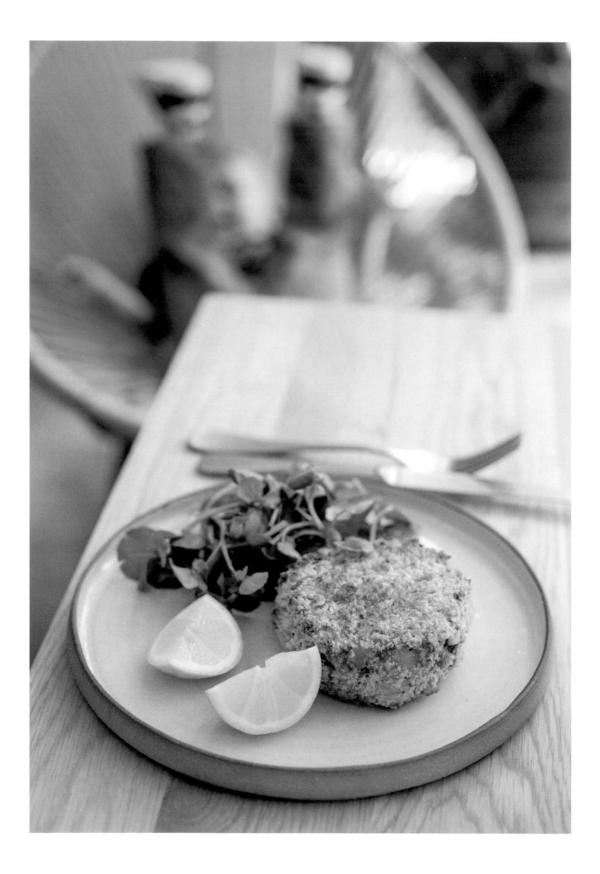

Baked tuna fish cakes

These are big, proper fish cakes that I'd be proud to serve up at my pub. Make sure you buy really good-quality tuna – it will make all the difference. Baking the potatoes first, rather than boiling them, keeps in the flavour and moisture so they are less likely to dry out as you cook the fish cakes.

Serves: 4

Calories: 345 per serving

4 medium baking potatoes (800g)
4 spring onions, finely sliced
50g gherkins, finely chopped
2 tbsp baby capers
2 tsp Dijon mustard
Finely grated zest of 1 lemon
A handful of flat-leaf parsley
    leaves, finely chopped
250g good-quality tinned albacore
    tuna (in spring water)
Olive oil spray
Sea salt and freshly ground
    black pepper

To coat
1 large free-range egg, beaten
70g dry white breadcrumbs
    (made from one-day old bread)

To serve
Lemon wedges
Watercress
Herb dressing (see page 186),
    optional

1. Preheat the oven to fan 200°C/gas 6. Cook the potatoes on a baking tray in the oven for 50 minutes to 1 hour, or until soft right through. Remove and set aside to cool. (Turn off the oven.)

2. Spoon out the potato flesh into a large bowl and mash it roughly. Add the spring onions, gherkins, capers, mustard, lemon zest and parsley. Season generously with salt and pepper and mix well. Drain the tuna, then gently fold it in, being careful not to break it up too much.

3. Divide the mixture into 4 portions and shape into patties. Chill in the fridge for at least 2 hours to firm up (overnight is fine).

4. When you're ready to cook the fish cakes, heat the oven to fan 200°C/gas 6. Line a baking tray with baking parchment and spray it with oil. Have the beaten egg and breadcrumbs ready in separate shallow bowls; season both with salt and pepper.

5. Coat each fish cake first in the beaten egg and then in the breadcrumbs, making sure they are coated all over. Place the fish cakes on the prepared tray and spray each one with oil. Cook for 15 minutes, then flip each fish cake over and cook for another 15 minutes.

6. Serve hot, with lemon wedges and watercress, dressed with herb dressing if you wish.

Soy-glazed salmon salad

Asian flavours add layers and complexity to this salad to keep your palate excited! Nori sheets are 100% natural toasted seaweed – low in fat, low in calories and about one-third protein – with an amazing umami flavour. They're great scrunched into Asian salads like this for extra taste and texture.

Serves: 4

Calories: 320 per serving

4 skinless salmon fillets
   (120g each)
Sunflower oil spray

For the marinade
2 tbsp light soy sauce
2 tbsp mushroom ketchup
1 tbsp Sriracha hot sauce
2 garlic cloves, finely grated
3cm piece of ginger, finely grated
1 tsp granulated sweetener

For the salad
100g Chinese cabbage, shredded
100g cucumber, julienned
100g kohlrabi, julienned
100g carrot, julienned
100g bean sprouts
A handful of coriander leaves,
   roughly chopped
Juice of 1 lime
1 tbsp light soy sauce

To serve
1 red chilli, finely sliced
8 crispy nori strips/thins
   (snack size)
A small handful of Asian
   micro-herbs

1. Mix the marinade ingredients together in a bowl. Add the salmon fillets and turn to coat. Cover and leave to marinate in the fridge for up to 2 hours.

2. Meanwhile, for the salad, toss all the ingredients together in a large bowl to combine.

3. When you're ready to cook your salmon, heat a medium non-stick frying pan over a very high heat. Spray with 6–10 sprays of oil. Lift the salmon into the pan, reserving the marinade, and cook, without moving, for 2–3 minutes. Flip the fillets over, turn down the heat to low and cook for 4–5 minutes on the other side. Transfer the salmon to a plate to rest.

4. Pour the marinade into the frying pan and let it bubble for a minute or so, until it reduces down to a glaze. Pour this over the resting salmon and leave for 3–4 minutes.

5. Divide the salad between four plates. Flake the salmon on top of the salad and trickle over any remaining soy glaze. Sprinkle with red chilli, torn nori sheets and micro-herbs.

THE LOWDOWN Don't let the salmon marinate for longer than 2 hours or the salt in the soy will start to cure it.

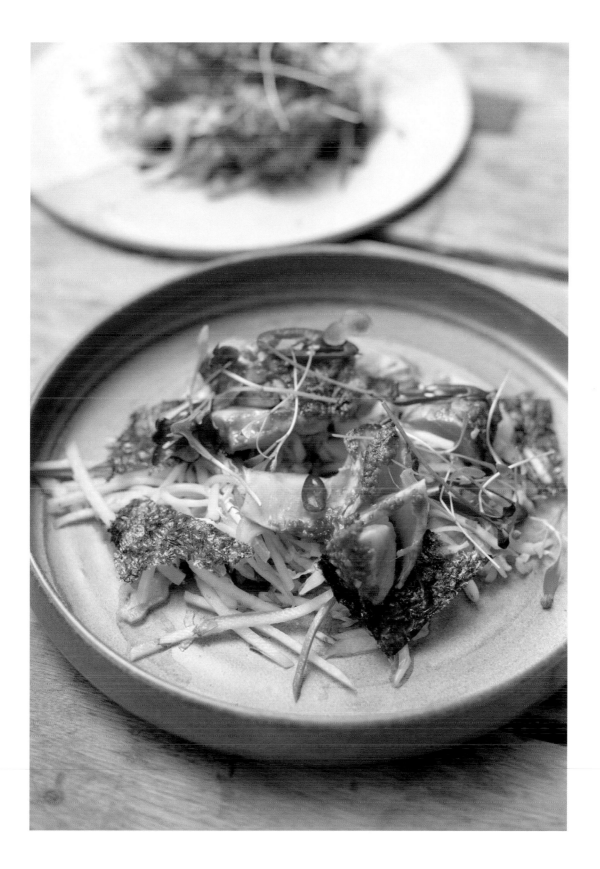

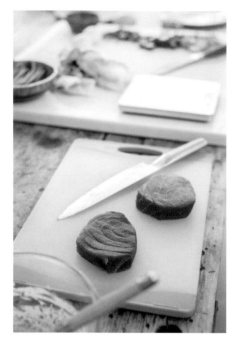

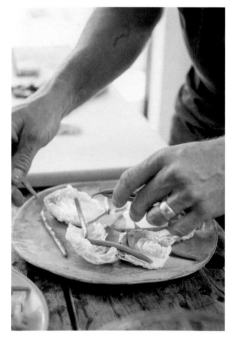

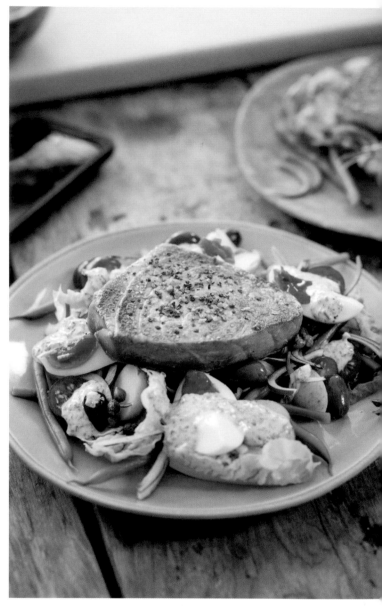

Tuna niçoise

The key to this recipe is to season the tuna generously and cook it over a high heat to give it an extra smoky, charred taste, taking care to avoid overcooking it. The dressing is another low-cal winner, heavy on the herbs and very low in fat. Try it with other salads, or drizzled over veggie dishes.

Serves: 2

Calories: 350 per serving

2 medium free-range eggs
150g fine green beans
2 little gem lettuce, leaves
    separated
100g baby new potatoes, boiled,
    cooled and halved (or quartered
    if large)
½ red onion, thinly sliced
100g cherry tomatoes, halved
25g pitted black olives
1 tsp baby capers
2 yellowfin tuna steaks
    (120g each)
Olive oil spray
Juice of ½ lemon
Sea salt and freshly ground
    black pepper

For the dressing
30g Greek yoghurt (0% fat)
1 tsp extra virgin olive oil
1 tsp water
1 tsp Dijon mustard
Finely grated zest and juice of
    ½ lemon
A pinch of golden caster sugar
½ tsp dried herbes de Provence
1 tbsp basil leaves, finely chopped
1 tbsp flat-leaf parsley leaves,
    finely chopped

1. Bring a small pan of water to the boil. Carefully lower in the eggs and cook for 6 minutes. Remove the eggs from the pan (but keep the water boiling) and place them in a bowl of cold water to cool.

2. Add the green beans to the pan with a pinch of salt and cook for 3–4 minutes. Drain the beans, run under cold water to cool, then drain thoroughly.

3. Arrange the lettuce leaves, new potatoes, green beans, red onion, tomatoes, olives and capers on two serving plates.

4. Heat a griddle or frying pan over a medium-high heat. Season both sides of the tuna generously with salt and pepper. Spray one side of each tuna steak with 5 sprays of oil and place, oiled side down, in the pan. Spray the top of each steak with 5 more sprays of oil. Cook for 1–2 minutes on each side; it should still be pink in the middle.

5. Remove from the heat and squeeze over the lemon juice, then lift the tuna out onto a plate and leave to rest for a couple of minutes.

6. Meanwhile, whisk all the dressing ingredients together in a small bowl. Shell the eggs and cut them into wedges.

7. Lay the boiled egg wedges on top of the salad, then add the tuna (breaking it into chunks first if you wish). Sprinkle with salt and pepper, drizzle over the dressing and serve.

Cajun prawn and kale salad

Heady Deep South spices work so well with prawns and chicken in a classic Louisiana gumbo dish. Richly flavoured kale, zingy lime and aromatic coriander give this lighter version a real vibrancy.

Serves: 2

Calories: 220 per serving

For the kale
100g kale leaves, roughly torn
Juice of 1 lime
1 tbsp extra virgin olive oil
Sea salt and freshly ground
    black pepper

For the Cajun prawns
220g raw tiger prawns, peeled and
    deveined, leaving the tail on
2 tsp Cajun spice mix
Olive oil spray
2 garlic cloves, finely chopped
½ Scotch Bonnet chilli,
    finely chopped
½ red pepper, cored, deseeded
    and sliced into strips
½ yellow pepper, cored, deseeded
    and sliced into strips
2 celery sticks, thinly sliced on
    an angle
2 medium-large tomatoes, diced
Juice of 1 lime
A handful of coriander leaves,
    finely chopped

1. Put the torn kale into a bowl and trickle over the lime juice and olive oil. Season with salt and pepper, then massage the kale gently for 2 minutes. Set aside.

2. Place the prawns in a separate bowl and sprinkle with the Cajun spice mix and a good pinch of salt. Toss to coat the prawns well. Heat a non-stick frying pan over a high heat. When hot, add 10 sprays of oil. Add the prawns and cook for 2–3 minutes, tossing frequently, or until they just turn pink. Remove from the pan and set aside.

3. Return the pan to the heat and add another 15 sprays of oil. Toss in the garlic, chilli and pepper strips and cook for 2–3 minutes, then add the celery and tomatoes and cook for 2 minutes.

4. Return the prawns to the pan, add the lime juice and cook for 2–3 minutes or until the prawns turn pink and are properly cooked through. Take the pan off the heat, stir through the coriander and season with salt and pepper to taste.

5. Spread the seasoned kale out on a large serving plate and top with the hot Cajun prawn mix. Serve straight away.

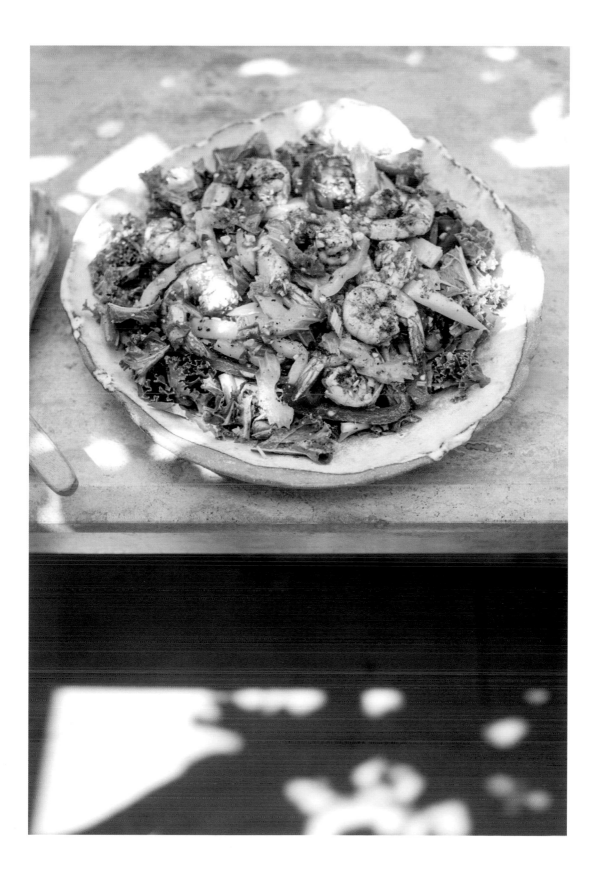

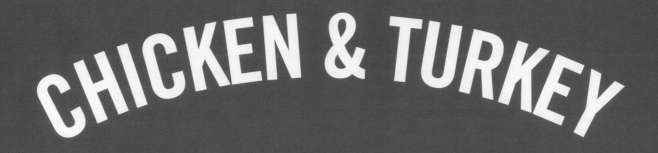

CHICKEN & TURKEY

It's important to keep mealtimes exciting, but it's also vital that you're able to stick with your diet long term. For this reason, I wanted to base the recipes in this book on everyday ingredients, so they can fit easily into your lifestyle. Chicken – and by extension turkey – is one of the most popular items in our shopping baskets. It's also a great choice for dieters because it is low in fat, especially if you remove the skin. So, I've devoted a whole chapter to these birds.

In several of the recipes in this chapter I poach a chicken crown in stock and then remove the meat from the bone. This keeps the meat lovely and succulent, and boosts the portion sizes – as shrinkage is kept to a minimum. Below are the basic instructions for poaching a crown. You can, if you like, use regular chicken breasts or thighs in any of the recipes in this chapter, but try using a crown and you'll see what a difference it makes to the finished dish.

Comfort eating is a major issue when it comes to dieting – one over-indulgent lapse can derail an entire week of hard work. I know just what it's like to want a big bowl of pasta or a juicy burger after a long day. You don't want to feel deprived because you are cutting down on calories, so I've come up with a low-calorie turkey take on spaghetti Bolognese (see page 130) and the diet-friendly burgers on page 120 use low-fat turkey mince instead of beef or lamb.

Being on a diet doesn't mean you can't enjoy a meal with your mates, and if you do the cooking you'll know exactly what you're eating. My Southern-style chicken thighs on page 135 are a real crowd-pleaser but they're baked not fried so they have much less fat. Get the gang round the table for a finger-licking feast!

TO POACH A CHICKEN CROWN

Place a 750g skinless chicken crown, breast side down, in a medium saucepan and cover with 500ml fresh chicken stock and 500ml cold water, topping up with more water if needed. Bring to a gentle simmer over a medium heat and cook for 20 minutes, then turn the chicken over and cook for a further 15 minutes. Turn off the heat and leave the chicken to cool in the stock. A 750g chicken crown will yield about 500g poached meat off the bone. Keep the stock, freezing any you don't need for the recipe (for up to 6 months) to use the next time you poach a crown, or for making soups or stews and casseroles.

Jerk chicken and tomato salad

This is such a lovely summertime dish. The punchy coating and seasoning brings it all to life and it has a really refreshing, cooling crunchy salad alongside to balance that fiery Caribbean heat.

Serves: 2

Calories: 240 per serving

For the jerk chicken
1 skinless chicken crown (750g), pre-poached in 500ml fresh chicken stock and 500ml water then cooled (see page 105)
2 tsp jerk seasoning
Sea salt and freshly ground black pepper

For the salad
80g mixed salad leaves
2 medium tomatoes, roughly chopped
2 baby cucumbers, sliced
½ red onion, thinly sliced
½ yellow pepper, cored, deseeded and thinly sliced

For the dressing
2 tbsp extra virgin olive oil
Juice of 1 lime
1 tsp runny honey
½ red chilli, deseeded and finely chopped
1 tbsp finely chopped coriander

1. Cut the cooked chicken breasts from the bone, place them on a metal tray and dust both sides with jerk seasoning and a little salt and pepper. Slice the breasts thickly on an angle, fanning them out slightly, and wave a cook's blowtorch over the surface until they are lightly charred.

2. Divide the salad leaves between two serving plates and scatter over the tomatoes, cucumber, red onion and yellow pepper.

3. For the dressing, whisk the ingredients together in a small bowl to combine.

4. Arrange the charred chicken breast slices on top of the salad, overlapping them slightly. Spoon over the dressing and serve.

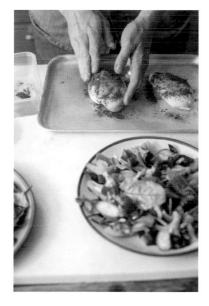

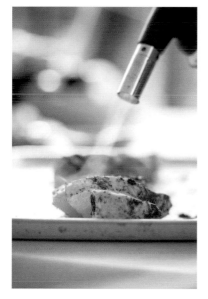

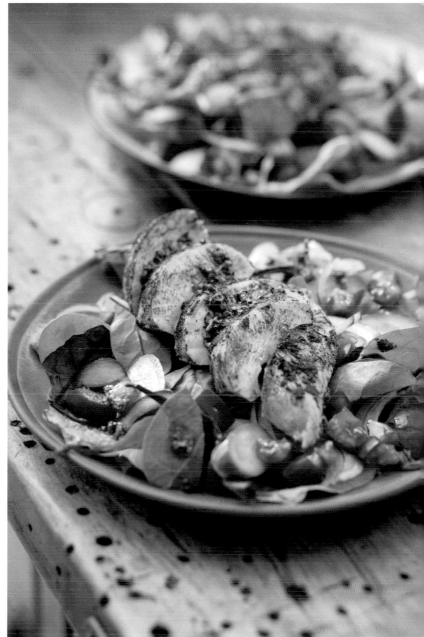

Chicken saltimbocca

Wrapping a chicken breast in Parma ham adds another layer of savoury flavour and keeps the meat inside lovely and tender. The tiniest amount of butter stirred through the sauce gives it a silky richness – a little goes a long way.

Serves: 2

Calories: 240 per serving

1 skinless chicken crown
  (about 800g)
500ml fresh chicken stock
500ml water
2 slices of Parma ham (30g in
  total)
8 sage leaves
1 tsp olive oil
2 tbsp Marsala wine
1 tsp cornflour, mixed to a paste
  with 1 tsp water
1 tsp butter
Sea salt and freshly ground
  black pepper
160g tenderstem broccoli,
  steamed, to serve

1. Place the chicken crown, breast side down, in a medium saucepan and pour on the stock and water. If it's not fully covered, top it up with more water. Bring to a gentle simmer over a medium heat and cook for 15 minutes, then turn the chicken over and cook for a further 10 minutes. Turn the heat off and leave the chicken to cool in the stock.

2. When cool, lift the chicken crown out of the stock. Using a sharp knife, cut the cooked breasts from the bone, keeping them whole. Reserve 150ml of the stock for the sauce. (Refrigerate the rest to use in another recipe; it will keep for 2–3 days.)

3. Season the cooled chicken breasts on both sides with salt and pepper. Lay the slices of Parma ham on your work surface and place two sage leaves on each one. Lay a chicken breast in the middle of the Parma ham, then top with two more sage leaves. Wrap the Parma ham around the chicken and seal to enclose.

4. Heat a medium non-stick frying pan over a high heat. Add the oil and cook the wrapped chicken breasts for 2–3 minutes on each side, or until nicely browned all over.

5. Take the pan off the heat and immediately add the Marsala; allow it to reduce by half, then pour in the reserved chicken stock. Return to the heat and simmer gently until the sauce has reduced slightly. Lift out the chicken breasts onto a plate and set aside to rest.

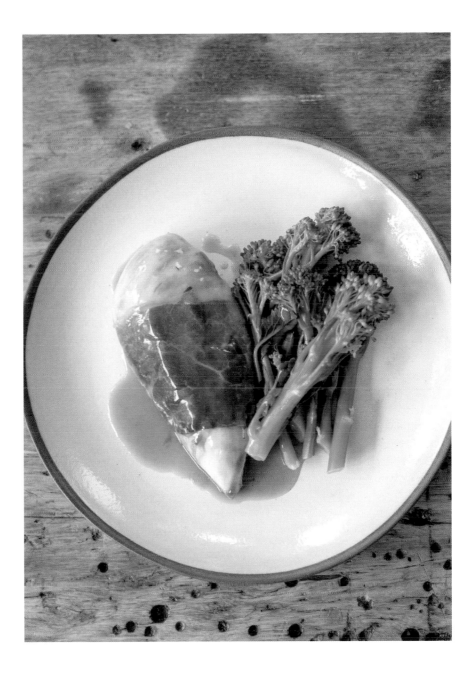

6. Stir the cornflour paste into the sauce and simmer, stirring, for 2 minutes or until thickened. Remove from the heat and stir in the butter, for a touch of richness.

7. Serve the chicken breasts with the sauce spooned over and steamed broccoli alongside.

Chicken casserole

This easy one-pot meal is a very simple version of *coq au vin* using chicken thighs, which are full of flavour. It has the added advantage that it can be cooked a day or two in advance and reheated to serve. My chicken crumble topping introduces an extra layer of taste and texture. You will have more than you need (enough for 8 servings); store the rest of the crumble in an airtight container (for up to 2 weeks) and sprinkle onto dishes that need a bit of extra flavour and crunch.

Serves: 4

Calories: 465 per serving
325 without crumble

8 large skinless, bone-in chicken thighs (670g in total)
200ml red wine
Olive oil spray
3 rashers of smoked back bacon (110g in total), cut into strips
200g baby onions, peeled
150g carrots, diced
100g celery, diced
3 sprigs of thyme
200g button mushrooms
300ml fresh chicken stock
2 tbsp cornflour, mixed to a paste with 2 tbsp water
A handful of flat-leaf parsley leaves, finely chopped
Sea salt and freshly ground black pepper

For the chicken crumble (optional)
30g bran flakes
10g millet flakes
2 tbsp dried onion flakes
1 crumbly chicken stock cube
3 tsp dried sage
½ tsp thyme leaves
3 tbsp flaked almonds, toasted and roughly chopped

1. Remove any excess fat from the chicken thighs. Put the chicken into a bowl, pour over the red wine and leave to marinate in the fridge overnight.

2. When you're ready to cook the chicken, preheat the oven to fan 180°C/gas 4.

3. Remove the chicken from the bowl and pat dry with kitchen paper, reserving the marinade. Spray each thigh 2 or 3 times with oil on each side.

4. Heat a large flameproof casserole over a high heat and sear the chicken thighs on both sides, until well browned. Remove from the pan and set aside.

5. Add the bacon strips to the pan and fry until crispy. Toss in the onions and carrots and sauté for 2–3 minutes. Add the celery, thyme, mushrooms, chicken and reserved marinade and bring to the boil. Pour in the chicken stock and bring to a simmer. Put the lid on and braise in the oven for 1 hour.

6. To make the chicken crumble, crush the bran, millet, onion flakes, stock cube, sage, thyme and ½ tsp salt to a coarse mixture, using a pestle and mortar. Dry-fry, stirring, in a small pan over a low heat for 2–3 minutes, until toasted and browned. Stir through the flaked almonds and leave to cool.

7. After an hour, remove the casserole from the oven and transfer the chicken pieces to a plate.

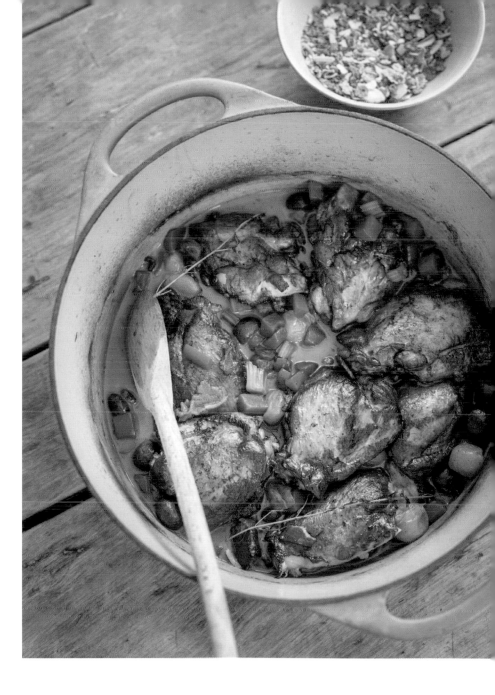

8. Place the casserole over a medium heat and stir in the cornflour paste. Stir for a couple of minutes until the sauce thickens. Season with salt and pepper and return the chicken to the casserole. Stir through the chopped parsley.

9. Serve in warmed bowls, sprinkled with the chicken crumble if using.

Chicken with peas, mushrooms and celeriac mash

This is such an indulgent and delicious meal that you won't feel like you're on a diet at all. With its fresh, clean flavour, celeriac makes a good counterbalance to the rich and sweet umami chicken; it's also lower in calories than mashed potato.

Serves: 4

Calories: 415 per serving

1 skinless chicken crown (750g),
    pre-poached in 500ml fresh
    chicken stock and 500ml water
    then cooled (see page 105)
40g dried porcini mushrooms
150ml boiling water
½ tbsp light olive oil
3 rashers of smoked back bacon
    (110g in total), cut into strips
2 banana shallots, finely diced
1 tbsp white wine vinegar
400ml fresh chicken stock
    (reserved from poaching
    the chicken)
300g button mushrooms, halved
150g frozen peas
2 tbsp cornflour, mixed to a paste
    with 2 tbsp water
A handful of flat-leaf parsley
    leaves, finely chopped
Sea salt and freshly ground
    black pepper

For the celeriac mash
1kg peeled and diced celeriac
    (1 medium-large)
4 tbsp semi-skimmed milk
1 tbsp low-fat vegetable spread

1. Have the poached chicken crown ready. Put the dried porcini in a small bowl, pour on the boiling water and leave to soak for 20 minutes.

2. For the mash, put the celeriac into a large pan, cover with water and add a generous pinch of salt. Bring to the boil, lower the heat and simmer for 15–20 minutes or until the celeriac is soft. Drain, then return the celeriac to the pan and mash well. Add the milk and vegetable spread; mash again. Season with salt and pepper to taste and set aside.

3. Heat a large non-stick saucepan over a high heat. Add the oil, then the bacon strips and cook for 3–4 minutes until browned and crispy. Add the shallots and cook for 3–4 minutes until softened.

4. Add the wine vinegar and let it bubble away, then pour in the stock and add the button mushrooms. Strain the porcini soaking liquor into the pan, then roughly chop the rehydrated porcini and add these too. Simmer for 5 minutes.

5. Take the chicken breasts off the bone and slice them thickly. Add to the pan along with the peas. Stir in the cornflour paste and cook, stirring, for 2 minutes or until the sauce has thickened. Season with salt and pepper to taste. Take the pan off the heat and stir through the chopped parsley.

6. Warm the celeriac mash over a low heat. Serve the chicken in bowls with the mash alongside.

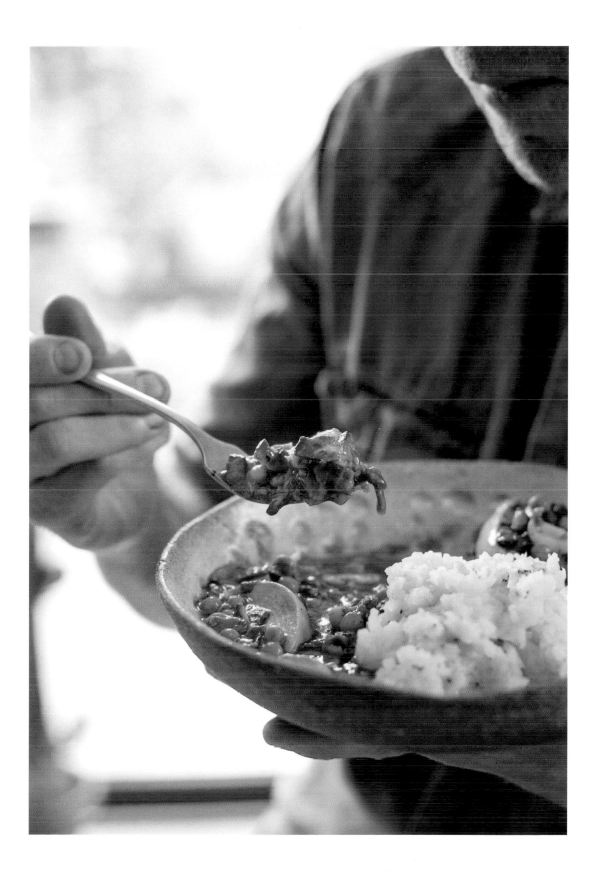

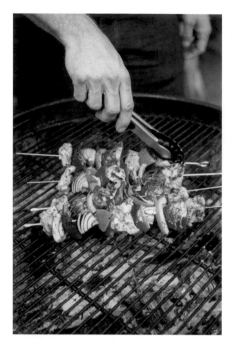
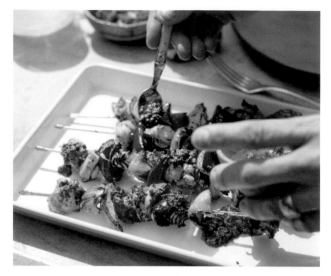
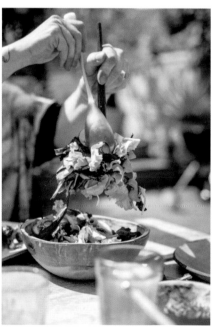
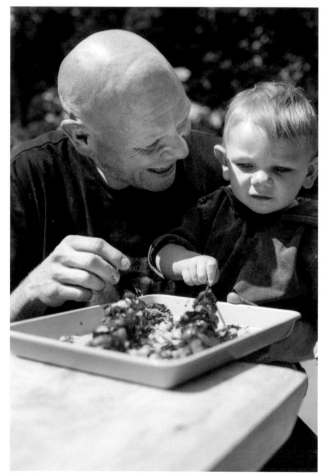

Greek kebabs

Greek kebabs are something I love to eat every time we go to Crete or Cyprus – two of my favourite holiday destinations. If the weather is good, you can conjure up those holiday vibes in your own back garden by whacking these kebabs on the barbecue to give them that authentic summery feel.

Serves: 4

Calories: 340 per serving

750g skinless, boneless chicken thighs, cut into 4cm pieces
2 tbsp finely chopped fresh oregano
4 garlic cloves, finely grated
Finely grated zest and juice of 1 lemon
1 tbsp extra virgin olive oil
1 large green pepper, cored, deseeded and cut into chunks
1 large red pepper, cored, deseeded and cut into chunks
2 beef tomatoes, halved and cut into wedges
1 red onion, cut into wedges
Olive oil spray
50g half-fat feta, crumbled
A handful of flat-leaf parsley leaves, finely chopped
Sea salt and freshly ground black pepper

For the dressing
1 tbsp extra virgin olive oil
1 tbsp red wine vinegar
1 tbsp water
20g pitted kalamata olives, finely chopped

1. Place the chicken pieces in a large bowl and add the oregano, garlic, lemon zest and juice, olive oil and some salt and pepper. Toss to coat the chicken then place in the fridge and leave to marinate for 1 hour.

2. Thread 3 pieces of chicken, 2 pieces each of green and red pepper, 2 tomato wedges and 2 onion wedges alternately onto each of 4 kebab skewers. Spray each skewer with a few sprays of oil.

3. Preheat the oven to fan 200°C/gas 6. Heat up your barbecue or a griddle pan over a high heat. Spray the griddle with a few sprays of oil. Cook the skewers on the barbecue or griddle for 5 minutes on each side, or until lightly charred.

4. Transfer the skewers to a baking tray and place in the oven for 10 minutes to finish cooking.

5. Meanwhile, for the dressing, in a small bowl, mix together the olive oil, wine vinegar, water and olives. Season with a little salt and pepper.

6. Transfer the cooked kebabs to a serving platter. Spoon over the dressing, crumble over the feta and sprinkle with parsley. Serve with a leafy salad.

THE LOWDOWN Removing the skin from chicken is a simple way to reduce fat and lower the calories.

Jerk chicken, cauliflower rice 'n' peas

Using cauliflower rice instead of actual rice is a clever swap when you're trying to cut back on calories. Cooking it in with the main dish allows it to take on all those delicious flavours. Packed full of fresh, filling ingredients, this is a really satisfying one-pan meal.

Serves: 4

Calories: 360 per serving

8 large skinless, bone-in chicken thighs (670g in total)
1 tbsp jerk seasoning
1 tsp flaky sea salt
Sunflower oil spray
1 large red onion, diced
1 large red pepper, cored, deseeded and diced
½ Scotch Bonnet chilli, deseeded and finely chopped
300g tomatoes, diced
500ml fresh chicken stock
400g tin kidney beans, rinsed and drained
600g cauliflower rice (see page 18)
2 handfuls of coriander leaves, roughly chopped
Sea salt and freshly ground black pepper

1. Remove any excess fat from the chicken thighs, then sprinkle both sides with the jerk seasoning and flaky salt.

2. Heat a large non-stick saucepan over a high heat. Spray each chicken thigh 2–3 times with oil and place in the pan, oiled side down. Spray the surface of the thighs with another 2–3 sprays of oil. Cook for 3 minutes on each side or until dark brown in colour (they won't be cooked all the way through at this stage). Depending on the size of your pan, you may need to do this in a couple of batches. Remove the chicken from the pan and set aside.

3. Add the onion to the saucepan and cook for 2 minutes, then toss in the red pepper and chilli and cook for another 2 minutes. Stir in the diced tomatoes and cook for 4–5 minutes or until they start to break down.

4. Pour in the chicken stock, stir and then cook for 10 minutes or until the liquor has reduced by one-third. Add the chicken thighs and cook for 10 minutes.

5. Add the kidney beans and cauliflower rice, stir through and cook for a further 10 minutes or until the cauliflower is tender. Season to taste and stir through some of the coriander.

6. Serve in warmed bowls, scattered with the rest of the chopped coriander.

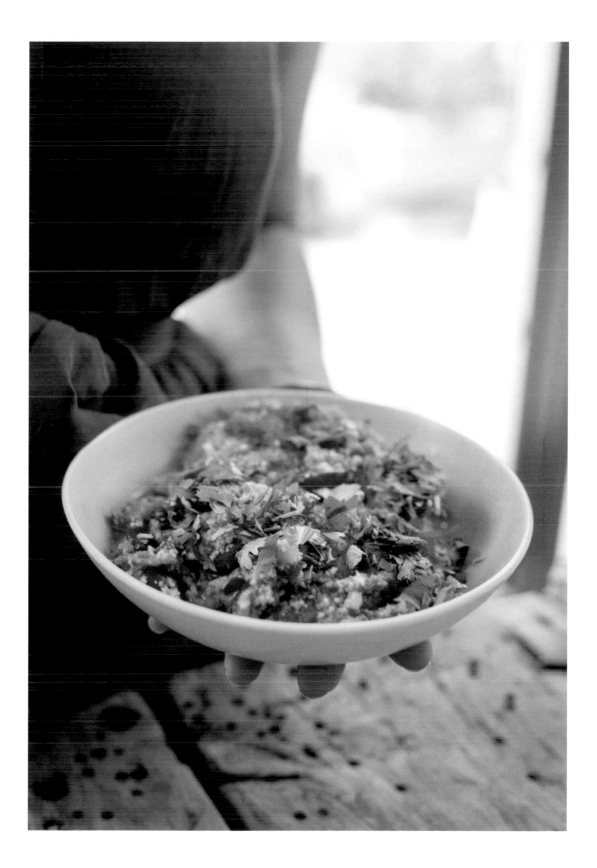

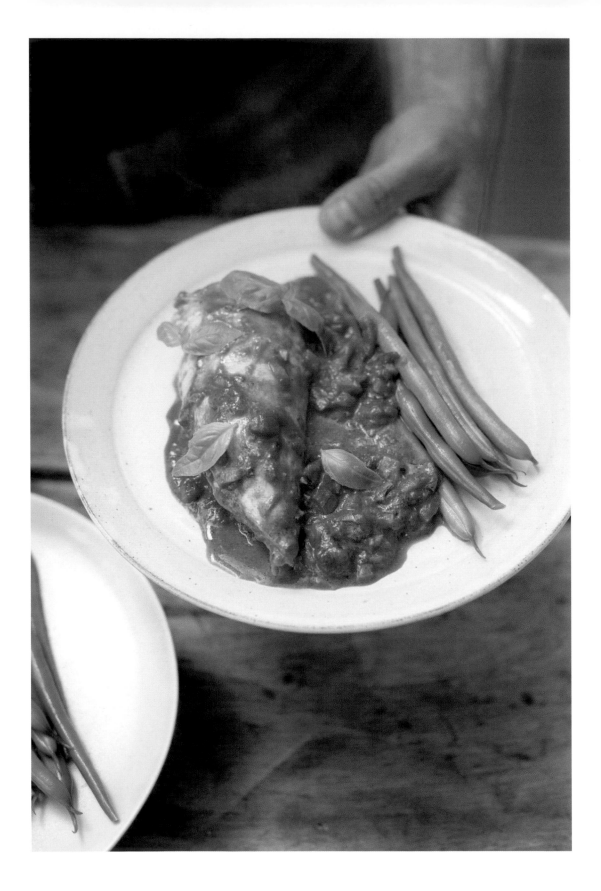

Chicken with tomato, mascarpone and basil

Low-fat mascarpone gives this Italian-style dish a beautiful, rich creaminess. Some people are averse to using tomatoes and mascarpone together but the combination works really well and is a great alternative to high-calorie butter or cream sauces.

Serves: 2

Calories: 355 per serving

1 skinless chicken crown (750g)
500ml fresh chicken stock
500ml water
1 tsp olive oil
½ onion, finely chopped
2 garlic cloves, finely chopped
1 tbsp tomato purée
400g tin chopped tomatoes
1 tbsp chopped fresh oregano
2 tbsp chopped basil, plus extra
    leaves to garnish
1 tsp aged balsamic vinegar
50g reduced-fat mascarpone
A pinch of dried chilli flakes
Sea salt and freshly ground
    black pepper
150g fine green beans, steamed,
    to serve

1. Place the chicken crown, breast side down, in a medium saucepan and pour on the stock and water. If it's not completely covered, top it up with more water. Bring up to a gentle simmer over a medium heat. Cook for 15 minutes, then turn the chicken over and cook for a further 10 minutes. Turn off the heat and leave the chicken to cool in the stock.

2. When cool, lift the chicken crown out of the pan; reserve 200ml of the stock. Using a sharp knife, carefully remove the cooked chicken breasts from the bone, keeping them whole.

3. Heat the oil in a frying pan over a medium heat. Add the onion and sauté for 5 minutes to soften, adding a splash of water if it starts to stick. Add the garlic and cook for 2 minutes. Stir in the tomato purée, chopped tomatoes, reserved chicken stock, oregano and some salt and pepper. Bring to a gentle simmer and cook for 10 minutes.

4. Add the chopped basil, balsamic vinegar and chicken breasts. Heat through for about 8 minutes on each side. Meanwhile, season the mascarpone with salt, pepper and chilli flakes, mixing well. Add to the pan and stir to combine with the sauce.

5. Transfer the chicken breasts to warmed plates and spoon on the sauce. Scatter with basil leaves and serve with steamed beans on the side.

Turkey and courgette burgers with mozzarella

I get how hard dieting can be – trust me, I've been right where you are. Sometimes a greasy burger smothered in cheese can be hard to resist. But stay strong! This lean turkey and mozzarella alternative tastes almost as good and it is so much better for you. Turkey is very low in fat but the grated courgette in the mix helps keep it moist.

Serves: 4

Calories: 605 per serving
345 without bun

500g turkey mince
500g grated courgette
2 tsp dried Italian herbs
2 tsp bicarbonate of soda
½ tsp dried chilli flakes
2 tbsp capers, roughly chopped
Olive oil spray
Sea salt and freshly ground
    black pepper

For the coleslaw
100g red cabbage, finely shredded
200g white cabbage, finely
    shredded
1 tsp salt
1 large carrot, grated
1 tsp toasted fennel seeds, ground
1 tbsp white wine vinegar
60g Greek yoghurt (0% fat)
2 tbsp half-fat mayonnaise

To serve
4 slices of half-fat mozzarella
    (30g each)
4 large wholemeal burger buns,
    toasted (optional)
4 thick slices of beef tomato
50g rocket leaves

1. Put the turkey mince into a large bowl. Take the grated courgette in handfuls and squeeze well to remove excess water, before adding to the bowl. Toss in the dried herbs, bicarbonate of soda, chilli flakes and capers, season with salt and pepper and mix well.

2. Divide the mixture into 4 equal portions and shape into burgers. Place on a baking tray lined with baking parchment and refrigerate while you make the slaw.

3. Put all the cabbage into a bowl, sprinkle with the salt and mix well. Leave to stand for 20 minutes, then rinse thoroughly and drain well. Mix in the other coleslaw ingredients.

4. Preheat the oven to fan 220°C/gas 7. Remove the tray of burgers from the fridge and spray each one with a couple of sprays of oil. Cook on the top shelf of the oven for about 12 minutes until golden brown and cooked through.

5. Lay a slice of mozzarella on each burger and cook for a further 4–5 minutes or until the cheese has melted.

6. Place a turkey burger inside each bun, if serving. Top with a slice of tomato and a handful of rocket leaves, then close the bun lids. Serve with the coleslaw on the side.

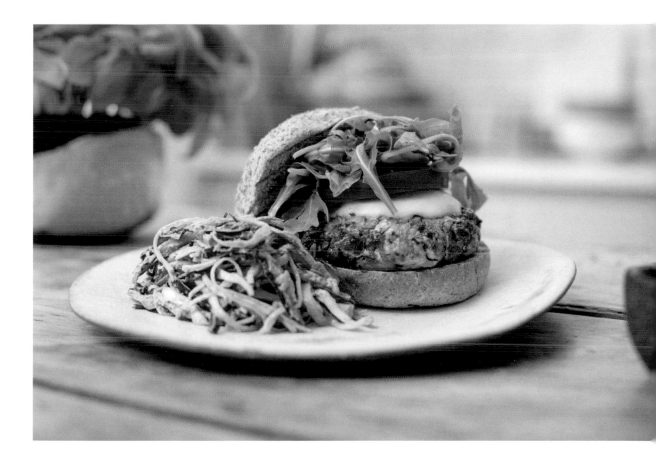

THE LOWDOWN Bicarbonate of soda is added to tenderise the meat and keep it juicy. Turkey can dry out quickly so it's worth adding a tenderiser such as this.

Chicken tikka masala

It may be Britain's favourite curry but grabbing a takeaway every week is a sure-fire way to pile on the pounds, as it's usually full of cream, oil and ghee. This is a lighter version that takes away the fat and calories, but still delivers on taste. Serving it with a raw Indian-style salad makes this an all-round fresh and delicious dish.

Serves: 4

Calories: 640 per serving
350 without rice

1 large skinless chicken crown
    (1kg)
Sea salt and freshly ground
    black pepper

For the marinade
Juice of ½ lemon
5cm piece of ginger, finely grated
4 large garlic cloves, grated
2 tbsp medium Madras curry
    powder
2 heaped tsp smoked paprika
A large pinch of salt
100g Greek yoghurt (0% fat)

For the curry sauce
1 tbsp sunflower oil
2 large onions, finely chopped
2 large garlic cloves, grated
2.5cm piece of ginger, finely grated
1 tsp ground turmeric
2 tsp paprika
2 tsp ground coriander
1 tbsp tomato purée
400g tin chopped tomatoes
300ml water
1 large red pepper, cored,
    deseeded and chopped
1 large green pepper, cored,
    deseeded and chopped
150g natural yoghurt (0% fat)
2 tbsp finely chopped coriander

1. Place the chicken in a large bowl or other non-reactive dish and slash the chicken breasts. For the marinade, mix all the ingredients together in a small bowl. Spread the marinade all over the crown. Cover with cling film and place in the fridge to marinate overnight, or for a minimum of 4 hours.

2. When you're ready to cook the chicken, preheat the oven to fan 120°C/gas ½. Place the marinated chicken in a roasting dish and spoon over any remaining marinade. Cook in the oven for 2 hours. (It won't be cooked right through at this stage.)

3. Meanwhile, make the curry sauce. Heat the oil in a large sauté pan. Toss in the onions and cook for 10 minutes or until they are golden brown, adding a splash of water to the pan if they begin to stick. Add the garlic and ginger with a splash of water, stir well and cook for 1 minute. Add the spices with some salt and pepper and cook for another minute.

4. Stir in the tomato purée and cook for a further minute, then tip in the tinned tomatoes and pour in the water. Bring to the boil, reduce the heat to a gentle simmer and cook for 5–10 minutes. Add the chopped peppers and cook for a further 5 minutes, then remove the pan from the heat.

5. Take the chicken out of the oven. Wave a cook's blowtorch over the surface until the marinade has slightly blackened in places. Set aside to rest for 10 minutes.

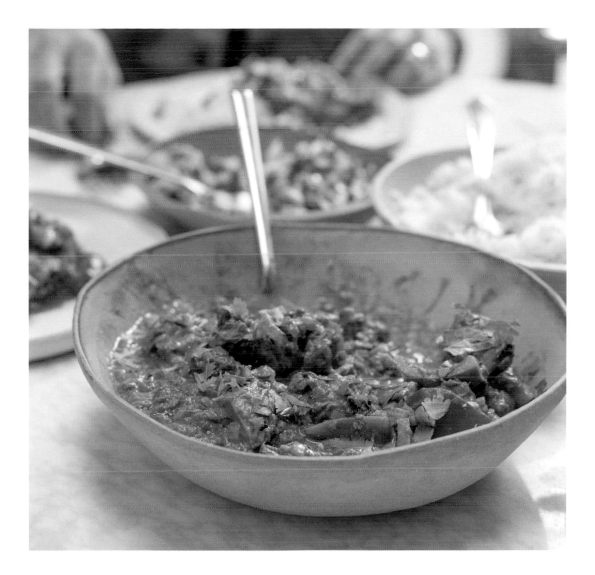

For the katchumber salad
1 small red onion, finely diced
2 large tomatoes, diced
⅓ cucumber (150g), diced
Juice of ½ lime
1 tsp chaat masala

To serve
Coriander leaves, roughly torn
320g basmati rice, cooked with salt and a pinch of saffron strands (optional)

6. For the katchumber salad, mix everything together in a bowl and set aside (no need to chill).

7. Take the chicken breasts off the bone and cut the meat into chunks, about 2.5cm. Reheat the curry sauce, then add the chicken and simmer for about 5 minutes, until the pieces are cooked through. Stir through the yoghurt and chopped coriander. Taste to check the seasoning.

8. Serve scattered with coriander, with saffron rice, if you like, and the katchumber salad alongside.

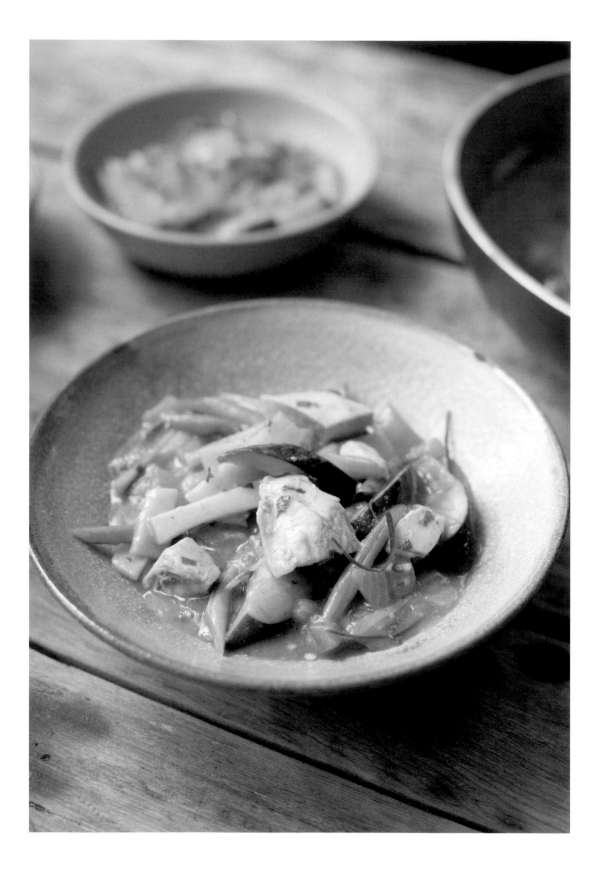

Thai green chicken curry

This is a tasty alternative to a takeaway, with plenty of interesting textures from the crunchy veg and bamboo shoots. The fiery ginger and Thai curry paste are perfectly balanced by the creamy, cooling coconut milk.

Serves: 4

Calories: 455 per serving

1 skinless chicken crown (750g), pre-poached in 500ml fresh chicken stock and 500ml water then cooled (see page 105)
1 tbsp vegetable oil
3 medium onions, cut into large dice
6 garlic cloves, finely chopped
7.5cm piece of ginger, julienned
4 tbsp good-quality Thai green curry paste (80g)
700ml fresh chicken stock (include the stock reserved from poaching the chicken)
100ml tinned full-fat coconut milk
1 tbsp fish sauce
1 tbsp oyster sauce
4 kaffir lime leaves, finely sliced
2 large green peppers, cored, deseeded and cut into large dice
200g fine green beans, halved
2 courgettes, cut into large dice
225g tin bamboo shoots, drained
3 heaped tbsp cornflour, mixed to a paste with 3 tbsp water
Chopped coriander, to finish (optional)

1. Take the chicken breasts off the bone and cut the meat into chunks, about 2.5cm.

2. Heat the oil in a large non-stick saucepan. When hot, add the onions and cook for 10 minutes or until they are softened and starting to brown, adding a splash of water if they start to stick.

3. Toss in the garlic and ginger and sauté for 2–3 minutes, then stir in the curry paste and cook, stirring frequently, for 2 minutes or until fragrant.

4. Add the chicken stock, coconut milk, fish sauce, oyster sauce and lime leaves. Bring to the boil and let the stock simmer for 5 minutes then toss in the peppers, green beans and courgettes, and cook for 5 minutes.

5. Add the chicken and bamboo shoots, then stir in the cornflour paste. Cook, stirring, for a couple of minutes until the liquor thickens.

6. Serve the curry in warmed big bowls, scattered with chopped coriander if you like.

Chicken satay

Satay sauce is usually high in calories but this is a lighter version using just enough agave to bring that lovely sweetness to the dish. Make sure you give the chicken enough time to marinate and absorb all the amazing bold flavours before you slow-roast it, which keeps it nice and moist.

Serves: 2

Calories: 235 per serving

1 skinless chicken crown (750g)

For the marinade
15g galangal root, finely chopped
2 lemongrass stems, finely sliced
1 tsp light soy sauce
1 tsp fish sauce
2cm piece of fresh turmeric root, chopped
1 long red chilli, sliced
1 shallot, chopped
Juice of 1 lime

For the satay sauce
1 tbsp crunchy peanut butter
1½ tbsp boiling water
1 tsp Sriracha hot sauce
½ tsp agave
1 tsp light soy sauce

To serve
120g cucumber, diced

1. For the marinade, blitz all the ingredients together in a small food processor until smooth.

2. Line a baking tray with baking parchment. Slash the breasts of the chicken crown and place on the lined tray. Spread the marinade over both sides of the chicken crown and rub into the slashes. Leave to marinate in the fridge for 4 hours, or overnight.

3. When you're ready to cook the chicken, preheat the oven to fan 100°C/gas ¼. Cook the chicken on the middle shelf for 1 hour, then remove. Increase the oven temperature to fan 220°C/gas 7.

4. When the oven is hot, roast the chicken crown on the top shelf for 30 minutes or until cooked through. Remove from the oven and wave a cook's blowtorch over the surface until charred and blackened in places. Leave to rest for 10 minutes.

5. Meanwhile, put the ingredients for the satay sauce in a small saucepan and bring to a simmer, stirring occasionally, then take off the heat.

6. Using a sharp knife, carefully remove the whole chicken breasts from the crown. Serve with the crunchy cucumber and satay sauce alongside.

THE LOWDOWN Marinating the chicken overnight ensures the meat will be beautifully tender, juicy and full of flavour.

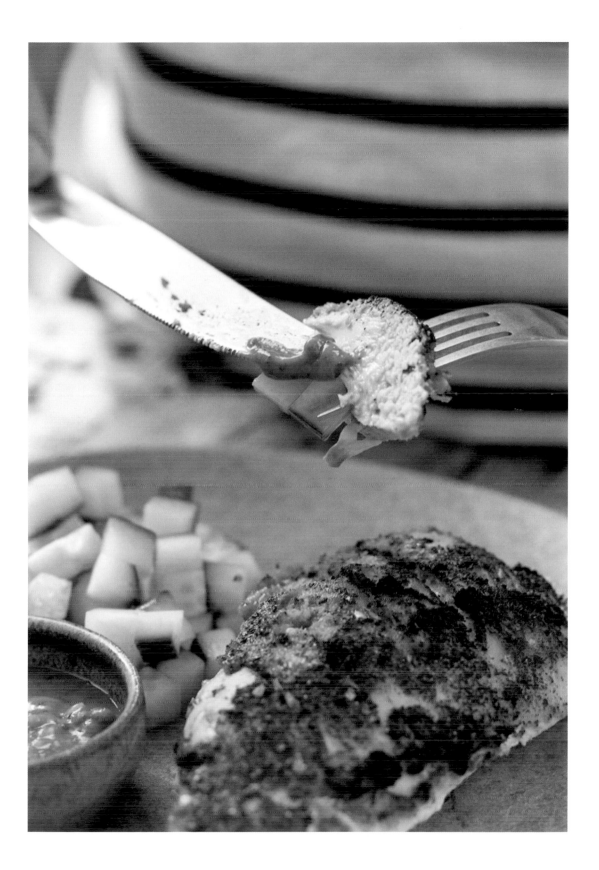

Chicken and mushroom filo crunch

Filo delivers a satisfying pastry crunch, which works so well with the rich umami mushroom filling in these moreish parcels. Dried mushrooms are huge on flavour so keep a tub on hand to enrich soups, stews and ragu sauces.

Serves: 6

Calories: 330 per serving

1 skinless chicken crown (650g)
500ml fresh chicken stock
500ml water
50g dried shiitake mushrooms
400ml just-boiled water
200g button mushrooms, halved
1 tbsp thyme leaves
6 spring onions, sliced
Finely grated zest of 1 lemon
1 tbsp cornflour
200g half-fat crème fraîche
1 tbsp liquid aminos
6 filo sheets
Olive oil spray
1 tsp nigella seeds
Sea salt and freshly ground
   black pepper

1. Place the chicken crown, breast side down, in a medium saucepan. Cover with stock and water, topping up with more water if needed, and bring to a gentle simmer over a medium heat. Cook for 15 minutes, then turn the chicken over and cook for a further 10 minutes. Turn off the heat and leave the chicken to cool in the stock.

2. Meanwhile, put the dried shiitake in a bowl, pour on the hot water and leave to soak for 20 minutes.

3. Strain the mushroom soaking liquor into a saucepan. Chop the rehydrated shiitake and add them to the pan, along with the button mushrooms and thyme. Bring to a gentle simmer and cook for 20 minutes or until the liquid has reduced to a glaze. Leave to cool.

4. Preheat the oven to fan 200°C/Gas 6. Line a baking tray with baking parchment. Lift the chicken out of the stock and pat dry with kitchen paper. Take the meat off the bone and cut into 2cm dice.

5. Place the diced chicken in a bowl with the cooled mushrooms, spring onions, lemon zest, cornflour, crème fraîche and liquid aminos. Mix together well and season with salt and pepper.

6. Divide the filling into 6 portions. Spray a sheet of filo lightly with oil, put a filling portion in the middle and shape it into a log. Wrap in the filo, folding the ends in to seal and form a parcel. Repeat with the rest of the filo and filling to make 6 parcels.

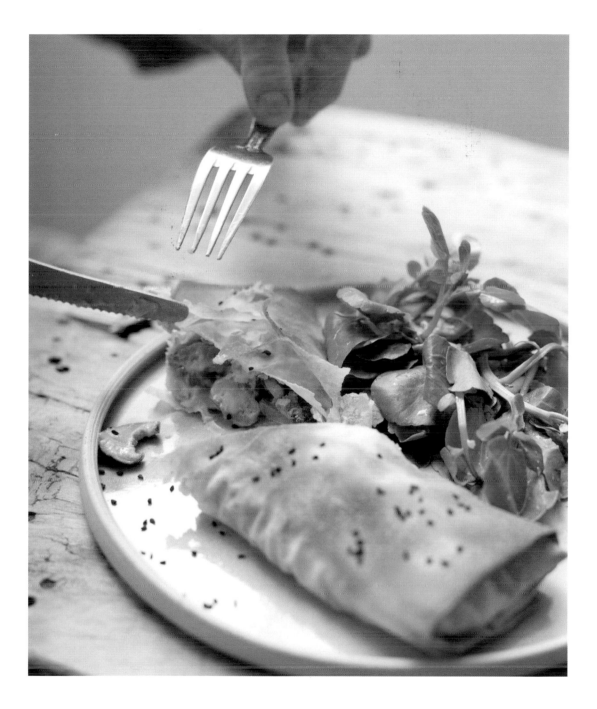

7. Place the filo rolls on the lined baking tray and spray the surface of each one with a little more oil. Sprinkle with black pepper and nigella seeds and bake in the oven for 20 minutes. Serve straight away, with a watercress salad on the side.

Turkey ragu with white cabbage linguine

This is basically a light version of spaghetti Bolognese using turkey mince, which is roasted for extra flavour and texture, and replacing pasta with tasty shredded cabbage linguine.

Serves: 4

Calories: 550 per serving

1kg turkey mince
1 tbsp light olive oil
2 large onions, finely diced
150g carrots, diced
100g celery, diced
6 garlic cloves, finely grated
2 tbsp caraway seeds
2 tbsp dried herbes de Provence
3 tbsp tomato purée
200ml red wine
2 x 400g tins chopped tomatoes
1.25 litres fresh chicken stock
600g white cabbage, cored and
    shredded into long, thin strips
120ml water
A handful of basil leaves,
    roughly chopped
Sea salt and freshly ground
    black pepper

THE LOWDOWN Salting the cabbage softens it slightly, yet it still retains a good level of crunch.

1. Preheat the oven to fan 180°C/Gas 4. Line a deep, lipped baking tray with baking parchment.

2. Spread the turkey mince out evenly on the lined baking tray and cook on the top shelf of the oven for 40 minutes, breaking it up well with a wooden spoon every 10 minutes. It should have a dark, even colour and resemble large coffee granules. Remove and set aside.

3. Heat the oil in a large non-stick saucepan over a medium heat. Add the onions and cook for about 10 minutes or until softened, then add the carrots and celery and cook for 5 minutes. Add the garlic and cook for another 2 minutes, then sprinkle in the caraway seeds and dried herbs. Cook for 1 minute, then add the tomato purée and cook, stirring, for another minute.

4. Pour in the red wine and let it bubble away. Add the tomatoes and chicken stock, bring to a simmer, then add the turkey to the pan. Simmer very gently for 45 minutes or until you have a thick ragu.

5. Meanwhile, put the cabbage into a large bowl, sprinkle liberally with salt and mix well with your hands. Leave for 20 minutes.

6. Rinse the cabbage thoroughly and drain well. Heat a non-stick pan over a medium heat. Add the cabbage with the water and stir until it wilts; drain.

7. Fold the basil through the turkey ragu and serve piled on top of the cabbage linguine.

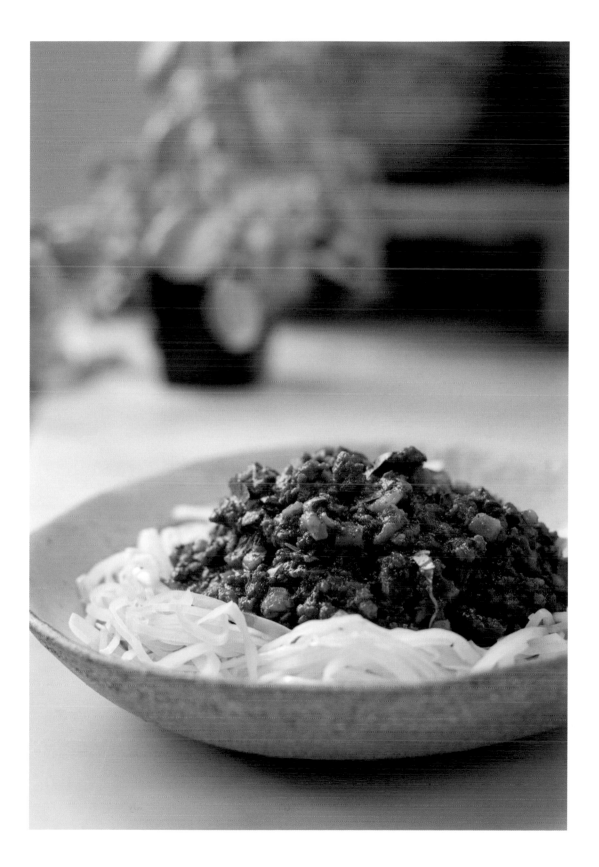

Chicken biryani

Replacing some of the rice in a classic biryani with cauliflower rice and a ton of veg means you get to eat a massive portion! Surely a total winner when you're watching the scales? Keep the chicken pieces chunky for an even more satisfying one-pot meal.

Serves: 4
Calories: 455 per serving

1 skinless chicken crown (650g)
500ml fresh chicken stock
500ml water
150g basmati rice
1 tbsp vegetable oil
2 large onions, finely chopped
4 garlic cloves, finely chopped
4cm piece of ginger, finely grated
A small handful of curry leaves
    (ideally fresh, but dried will do)
2 pinches of saffron strands
2 tbsp medium Madras curry
    powder
1 tbsp garam masala
1 tsp flaky sea salt
200g tomatoes, diced
200g carrots, finely diced
200g green beans, finely sliced
200g cauliflower, grated
Sea salt and freshly ground
    black pepper
Coriander leaves, roughly chopped,
    to serve

1. Place the chicken crown, breast side down, in a medium saucepan. Cover with the stock and water, topping up with more water if needed, and bring to a gentle simmer over a medium heat. Cook for 15 minutes, then turn the chicken over and cook for a further 10 minutes. Turn off the heat and leave the chicken to cool in the stock.

2. When cool, lift the chicken crown out of the pan and take the meat off the bone. Cut the chicken into large cubes, about 3.5cm, and reserve 750ml of the stock. Set aside.

3. Meanwhile, put the rice into a bowl, fill it with water and swish the rice around with your hands to release the starch. Drain the rice and repeat the process twice more, or until the water is clear and the starch is removed. Drain and set aside.

4. Heat a large non-stick saucepan over a high heat. Add the oil, followed by the onions and sauté for 5 minutes or until softened, adding a splash of water if they start to stick. Add the garlic, ginger and curry leaves and cook for a further 2 minutes.

5. Turn the heat down to medium-low and stir in the saffron, curry powder, garam masala and salt. Cook, stirring, for 1 minute, then add the tomatoes and cook for a further 2 minutes. Now add the rice, carrots, reserved chicken stock and some salt and pepper. Bring to a gentle simmer, cover and cook for 10 minutes. Remove the lid and stir well.

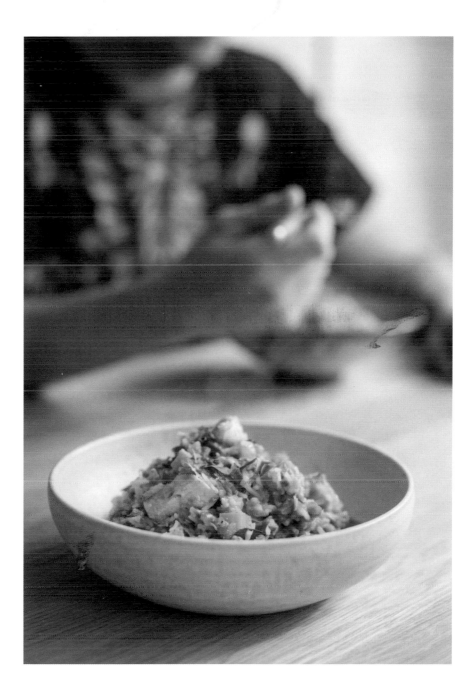

6. Add the chicken, green beans and cauliflower, stir gently to combine and put the lid back on. Cook at a low simmer for 8–10 minutes, or until the rice is cooked and the liquor has reduced down. The beans should retain a slight crunch. Serve in warmed bowls, scattered with coriander.

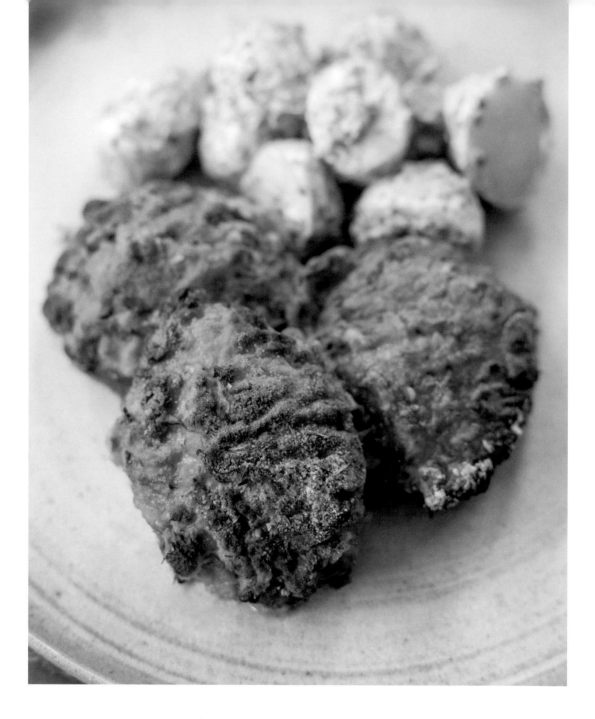

THE LOWDOWN A good potato salad is versatile – perfect for barbecues and with salads and cold meats. This one swaps high-calorie mayo for a delicious herby dressing, made with low-fat mayo and 0% fat Greek yoghurt.

Southern-style chicken with potato salad

Everybody likes fried chicken! This version has all the flavour you associate with fried chicken but much less fat because it is baked not fried. Put the chicken to marinate a day ahead if you can, so it becomes really juicy. The low-fat herby potato salad is a great accompaniment.

Serves: 4

Calories: 510 per serving
385 without potato salad

12 boneless, skinless chicken
    thighs (1kg in total)
75g plain flour
1 tsp garlic salt
1 heaped tsp smoked paprika
1 tsp dried thyme
Sunflower oil spray
Flaky sea salt and freshly ground
    black pepper

For the marinade
200ml low-fat buttermilk
1 tbsp Worcestershire sauce
½ tsp freshly ground black pepper
1 tsp flaky sea salt
½ tsp onion powder
½ tsp dried thyme
½ tsp dried oregano
½ tsp dried sage
¼ tsp white pepper

For the herby potato salad
600g new potatoes
2 tbsp Greek yoghurt (0% fat)
1 heaped tsp low-fat mayonnaise
1 tsp Dijon mustard
1 tsp white wine vinegar
40g cornichons, finely chopped
2 tbsp each finely chopped chives,
    flat-leaf parsley and mint

1. Remove any excess fat from the chicken thighs. Mix the marinade ingredients together in a large bowl, add the chicken and turn to coat. Place in the fridge to marinate overnight, or for at least 4 hours.

2. For the salad, put the new potatoes into a pan of cold water, bring to the boil and cook for about 20 minutes, until tender; drain. Leave to cool. In a small bowl, mix the yoghurt, mayonnaise, mustard and wine vinegar together.

3. When you're ready to cook the chicken, preheat the oven to fan 240°C/Gas 10. Line a large baking tray with baking parchment.

4. Mix the flour, garlic salt, smoked paprika, thyme and 1 tsp each flaky salt and ground black pepper together in a shallow bowl. Dip each marinated chicken piece into the flour mix and turn to coat well on all sides. Place on the lined baking tray.

5. Spray each piece of chicken 4 or 5 times with the spray oil. Cook on the top shelf of the oven for 20–30 minutes or until crispy, browned and cooked through. To test, poke the thickest part of the thigh with a skewer the juices should run clear.

6. To assemble the salad, halve the cooled potatoes and place them in a serving bowl. Add the yoghurt dressing and turn to coat, then stir through the rest of the ingredients, adding salt and pepper to taste. Serve with the hot Southern-style chicken thighs.

Piri piri chicken with pickled radishes

This is *hot, hot, hot!* It makes a great spicy alternative to a simple roast chicken, so why not have it instead of your traditional Sunday lunch? You will need to begin the day before in order to pickle the radishes and marinate the chicken.

Serves: 4

Calories: 375 per serving

---

1 skinless whole chicken (2kg)

For the piri piri sauce
4 long red dried chillies
100ml red wine vinegar
1 large red pepper
5 long red chillies,
**   roughly chopped**
6 garlic cloves, sliced
2 tsp hot smoked paprika
1 tsp dried oregano
1 tsp dried thyme
2 tsp flaky sea salt
1 tsp granulated sweetener
Juice of 2 lemons

For the pickled radishes
200g radishes, halved
1 tbsp flaky sea salt
2 star anise
1 tsp coriander seeds
200ml red wine vinegar
1 tbsp granulated sweetener

To serve (optional)
Lettuce with citrus dressing
**   (see page 152)**

1. First prepare the radishes, put them into a bowl, sprinkle with the salt and leave to stand for 2 hours. Wash off the salt and drain well. Put the star anise, coriander seeds, wine vinegar and sweetener into a small pan. Bring to a gentle simmer over a medium heat, then pour over the radishes. Leave to cool, then place in the fridge to pickle overnight.

2. To make the piri piri sauce, put the dried chillies and wine vinegar into a small saucepan, bring to a simmer then turn off the heat. Leave to stand for 15 minutes to rehydrate the chillies.

3. Meanwhile, spear the stalk of the red pepper with a fork and turn the pepper over the flame of a gas hob (or use a cook's blowtorch) until blistered and blackened all over. Place in a small bowl, cover with cling film and leave for 5 minutes.

4. Put the remaining sauce ingredients into a food processor with the wine vinegar and rehydrated chillies. Uncover the red pepper and remove all the skin and seeds. Add the pepper flesh to the processor and blitz thoroughly – it will be quite a loose mixture but you don't want any large bits.

5. Put the chicken into a large bowl or non-reactive dish and score all over (including the underside and legs), making the cuts about 1cm deep and 2.5cm apart. Pour the piri piri sauce over the chicken and massage well. Cover with cling film and leave to marinate in the fridge for at least 4 hours, ideally overnight.

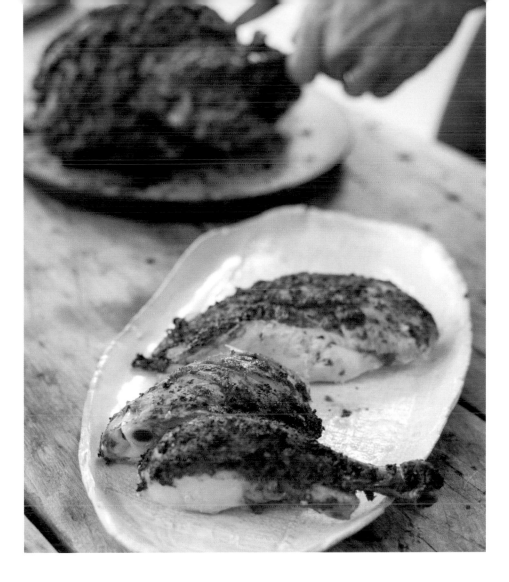

THE LOWDOWN Scoring the chicken before cooking ensures that the piri piri flavour goes *into* the meat not just on the outside.

6. When you're ready to cook the chicken, remove the cling film and leave at room temperature for an hour. Preheat the oven to fan 100°C/Gas ¼.

7. Place the chicken in a roasting tray and cook in the oven for 1½ hours. Remove and baste well with the sauce. Turn the oven up to fan 220°C/Gas 7. When it is hot, roast the chicken for 40–45 minutes. Remove and rest, covered with foil, for 10 minutes.

8. Carve the chicken and serve with the pickled radishes, and a salad of lettuce with citrus dressing (see page 152) for a cooling contrast if you like.

Chicken with fennel, garlic and tomatoes

This traybake is full of big Mediterranean flavours from the fennel, garlic and rosemary. Don't be put off by the huge amount of garlic – it mellows and sweetens beautifully as it roasts. Cooking the chicken low and slow keeps it deliciously moist without shrinkage, so the portions are satisfyingly substantial.

Serves: 3–4

Calories: 580–435 per serving

1 whole chicken (1.75kg)
1 large red onion, cut into
    6 wedges
1 large brown onion, cut into
    6 wedges
2 fennel bulbs, cut into thick
    wedges
20 garlic cloves, peeled but
    left whole
4 sprigs of rosemary, leaves
    stripped and finely chopped
200ml fresh chicken stock
Olive oil spray
200g cherry tomatoes on the vine
½ tsp onion powder
¼ tsp paprika
Sea salt and freshly ground
    black pepper

1. Preheat the oven to fan 120°C/Gas ½.

2. Place the chicken in a roasting tray and cook in the oven for 2 hours. (It won't be cooked through at this stage.) Remove from the oven and allow to rest for 30 minutes. Increase the oven temperature to fan 220°C/Fan 7.

3. While the oven is heating up, lay the onions, fennel and garlic in another roasting tray. Sprinkle with half the rosemary and season with salt and pepper. Pour on half the chicken stock and spray the veg 20 times with oil. Cook on the top shelf of the oven for 15 minutes.

4. Meanwhile, remove all the skin from the chicken and joint into 6 pieces. Remove the backbone but keep the ribcage in place on the two breast pieces. Blowtorch the chicken until lightly charred.

5. Remove the roasted veg from the oven and nestle the chicken pieces into the tray. Add the cherry tomatoes and pour on the remaining chicken stock. Sprinkle over the onion powder, paprika and the rest of the rosemary.

6. Spray each piece of chicken 4 times with oil and season with a little more salt and pepper. Return to the oven and bake for a further 20 minutes or until the chicken pieces are cooked through. To test, insert a skewer into the thickest part – the juices should run clear. Serve straight from the tray.

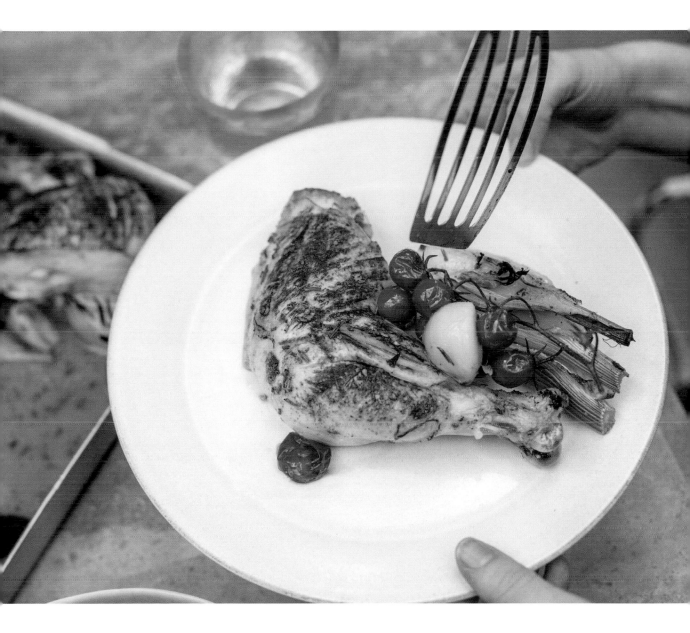

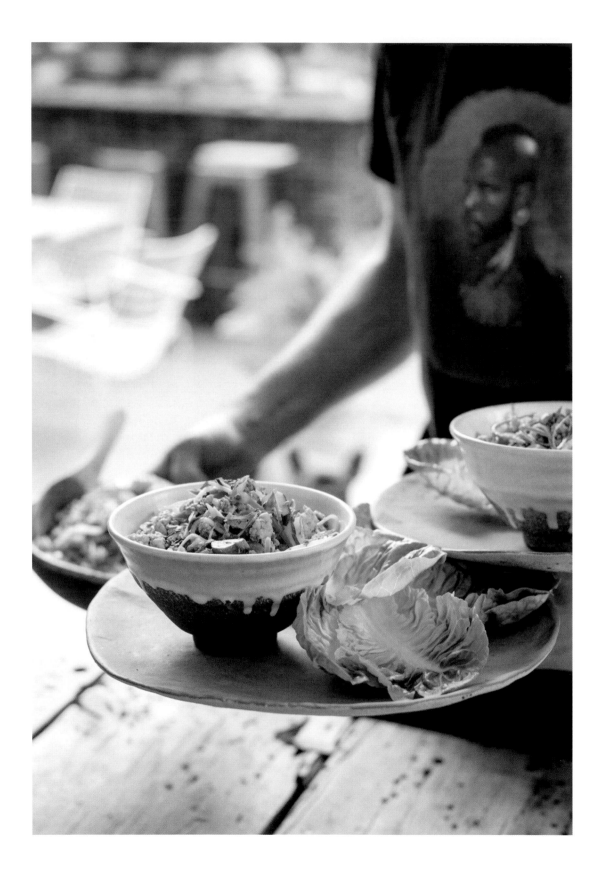

Turkey san choy bow

This super-tasty dish, packed with Asian flavours, is usually made with beef or pork but this version uses turkey mince, which is lower in fat. Lettuce leaf cups keep it low in cals and provide a cooling crunch alongside the salty spiced meal.

Serves: 4

Calories: 260 per serving

1 tbsp vegetable oil
½ onion, finely sliced
2 garlic cloves, finely chopped
2.5cm piece of ginger, finely grated
1 red chilli, finely chopped
500g turkey mince
1 large carrot, julienned
1 courgette, julienned
125g baby chestnut mushrooms, quartered
75g tinned water chestnuts, sliced
2 tbsp light soy sauce
1 tbsp oyster sauce
2 tbsp rice wine vinegar
100g bean sprouts
6 spring onions, finely sliced on an angle
A handful of coriander leaves, chopped
4 baby gem lettuce, leaves separated

1. Heat a large non-stick wok over a high heat and add the oil. When it is very hot, add the onion, garlic, ginger and chilli and cook for 1–2 minutes.

2. Add the turkey mince to the wok and stir-fry for 5–10 minutes, until it is just starting to brown, breaking up the mince with a wooden spoon as it cooks.

3. Toss in the carrot, courgette, mushrooms and water chestnuts and stir-fry for another 2 minutes. Add the soy sauce, oyster sauce and rice wine vinegar and cook for 2 minutes or until the liquor has bubbled away.

4. Stir through the bean sprouts, spring onions and chopped coriander and take off the heat.

5. Serve with the little gem leaves alongside to use as lettuce cups.

MEAT

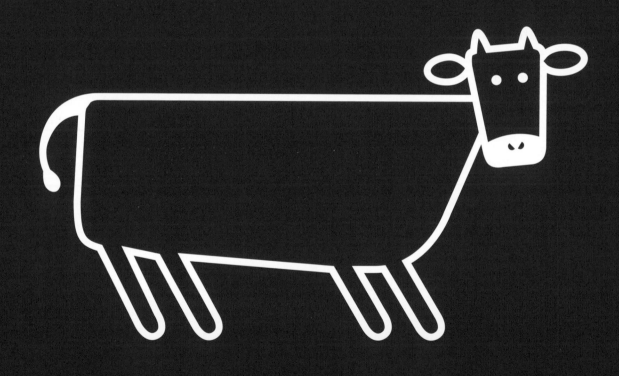

There is little doubt that takeaways and ready meals are a contributing factor to nationwide weight gain. Over 100 million are eaten each week in Britain and many are high in calories. But let's be honest: kebabs, curries and burgers are lush! So in this chapter I've created home-made versions of many fast food favourites, with all the flavour but fewer calories.

Meat can be tricky when you're on a diet, as it's often quite high in fat (and calories). But it is still possible to enjoy meat, you just have to look for ways of making it leaner wherever you can. Trim off the fat, use lean mince and choose cuts that are naturally lower in fat, such as tenderloin, topside and rump steaks.

If you're cutting down on fat, you'll also need to think a bit cleverly about how to avoid losing out on the flavour you usually get from roasting and frying. Cooking low and slow is one of my favourite options. The lengthy cooking time allows meat to become really succulent and tender, while the flavours work deep into the meat – try the Pot-roast topside of beef (page 156) or Pulled pork tacos (page 172) and you'll see what I mean.

Marinades and rubs are another great way of introducing intense flavour. The soy and ginger marinade applied to the Japanese-style pork tenderloin on page 166 elevates this dish to something special, and the spicy rub used on the roast beef for the salad on page 146 is incredibly punchy, giving the meat a fantastic flavour. When spices and seasonings work as hard as they do in these recipes, you often don't need quite as much meat on your plate to feel as though you've eaten something really substantial.

I look for ways to add flavour at every stage when I'm cooking. Roasting mince before you use it in a dish is an easy way of doing this – and you can drain off any fat once it's cooked, making it even leaner. Try the Spicy lamb mince curry (page 160), One-layer lasagne (page 152) and the Pork samosa pie (page 168). The additional cooking stage is well worth the effort – you can even pre-roast the mince a day ahead and keep it in the fridge.

I don't subscribe to the idea of making smaller portions when you're counting calories, because to stick to your diet you need to feel satisfied at every meal, and bulking up meat with other ingredients is a great way of making it go that little bit further – try the Spicy Moroccan lamb burgers (page 165), which have plenty of grated carrot and courgette added to the lean mince to keep the burgers lovely and moist as they cook.

Many of the recipes in this chapter are ideal for sharing, so try serving them in place of your Sunday roast – no one will realise they're tucking into diet food. I'll even bet some of these tasty meat dishes will become new family favourites.

Beef stroganoff

This lighter version uses half-fat crème fraîche instead of double cream but doesn't skimp on taste. It is finished with parsley, chervil and dried onion flakes for extra flavour and a bit of crunch.

Serves: 2

Calories: 795 per serving
505 without rice

½ tbsp light olive oil
1 large onion, finely sliced
3 garlic cloves, finely chopped
1 crumbly beef stock cube
2 tsp sweet smoked paprika
1 tbsp tomato purée
400ml tin beef consommé
150g baby chestnut mushrooms, thinly sliced
1 tbsp Dijon mustard
2 rump steaks trimmed of all fat (175g each)
Olive oil spray
60g cornichons, sliced
75ml half-fat crème fraîche
2 tbsp finely chopped flat-leaf parsley
2 tbsp chopped chervil
2 tbsp dried onion flakes
Sea salt and freshly ground black pepper

To serve (optional)
160g basmati rice, cooked

1. Heat the light olive oil in a large non-stick sauté pan over a low-medium heat. Add the onion and cook gently for 10 minutes or until softened and starting to caramelise.

2. Stir in the garlic and cook gently for 2 minutes. Crumble in the stock cube and stir in the paprika and tomato purée. Cook, stirring, for 2 minutes. Add the beef consommé, mushrooms and mustard. Bring to the boil, lower the heat and simmer for 10–15 minutes, until reduced by half.

3. Meanwhile, place a griddle pan over a high heat. Bash the steaks between two sheets of cling film, until about 5mm thick, then spray each on one side with 6 sprays of oil and season with salt and pepper. When the griddle is smoking hot, add the steaks and cook for 1 minute on each side. Remove and set aside to rest.

4. Once the sauce has reduced, remove from the heat and stir through the cornichons, crème fraîche, and most of the parsley and chervil (reserving some for garnishing). Stir in the juices from the resting meat and check the seasoning. Slice the meat into thick slices and stir into the sauce.

5. Mix together the dried onion flakes and reserved chopped parsley and chervil. Serve the stroganoff sprinkled with the onion and herb mix, with the rice on the side if you like.

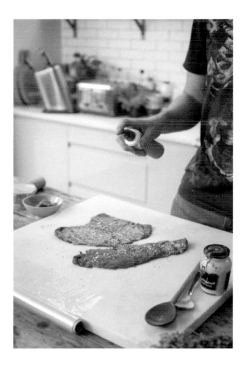
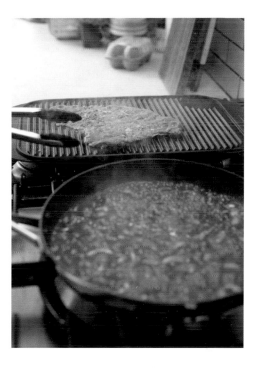
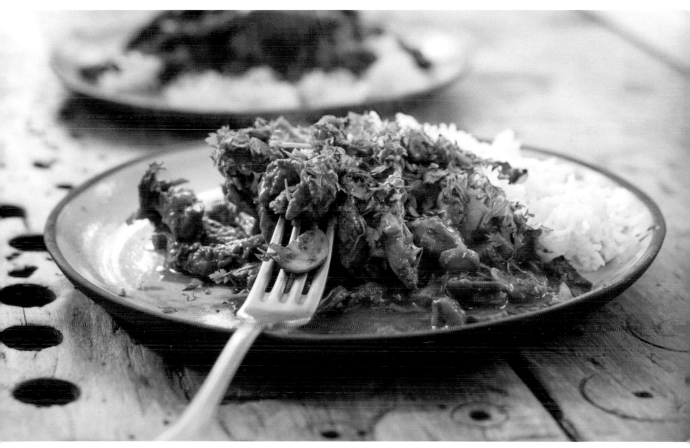

Roast beef salad with chimichurri sauce

This is a delicious way to enjoy roast beef, without the high-calorie extras it is usually served with. The low-cal version of fresh, herby chimichurri sauce balances the richness of the meat beautifully; it also goes well with grilled steak, chicken or fish.

Serves: 6

Calories: 290 per serving
245 without crumble

1kg joint of lean topside of beef (i.e. surface fat layer removed), rolled and tied
2 tsp flaky sea salt
1½ tsp coarse ground black pepper
2 tsp hot smoked paprika

For the beef crumble (optional)
35g crispbread
1 crumbly beef stock cube
½ tsp dried tarragon
40g biltong, roughly chopped
1 tbsp dried onion flakes
½ tsp salt

For the salad
130g watercress, rocket and spinach salad
2 little gem lettuce, quartered
5 tomatoes, cut into wedges
1 red onion, thinly sliced

For the chimichurri sauce
2 tsp finely chopped fresh oregano
2 tbsp finely chopped flat-leaf parsley
½ tsp dried oregano
½ tsp ground cumin
½ garlic clove, finely grated
1 heaped tsp Dijon mustard
1 red chilli, deseeded and finely chopped
2 tbsp extra virgin olive oil
2 tbsp sherry vinegar
2 tbsp water

1. Preheat the oven to fan 60°C/lowest gas.

2. Place the meat in a roasting dish. Mix together the salt, pepper and paprika and rub all over the beef. Cook in the oven for 4–5 hours, checking with a meat thermometer that the internal temperature has reached 58°C before removing. Leave to rest for 20 minutes. Use a blowtorch, if you like, to brown any areas of the meat that haven't coloured as well.

3. Meanwhile, for the crumble, in a small food processor, blitz the crispbread and stock cube for 10–20 seconds to reduce to crumbs. Tip into a small, dry pan and toast, stirring or shaking the pan, over a medium heat for 5 minutes. Set aside to cool, then add the rest of the ingredients.

4. Combine all the salad ingredients and divide between serving plates. For the chimichurri sauce, whisk all the ingredients together, seasoning with salt and pepper to taste.

5. Slice the beef thinly and lay on top of the salad then spoon over the sauce. Sprinkle with the savoury crumble, if using, then serve.

....

THE LOWDOWN My beef 'crumble' is a clever way of adding an extra layer of intense meaty flavour and crunch; you'll have more than you need (enough for 8–10 servings) so save the rest to use on salads, meat dishes or soups.

....

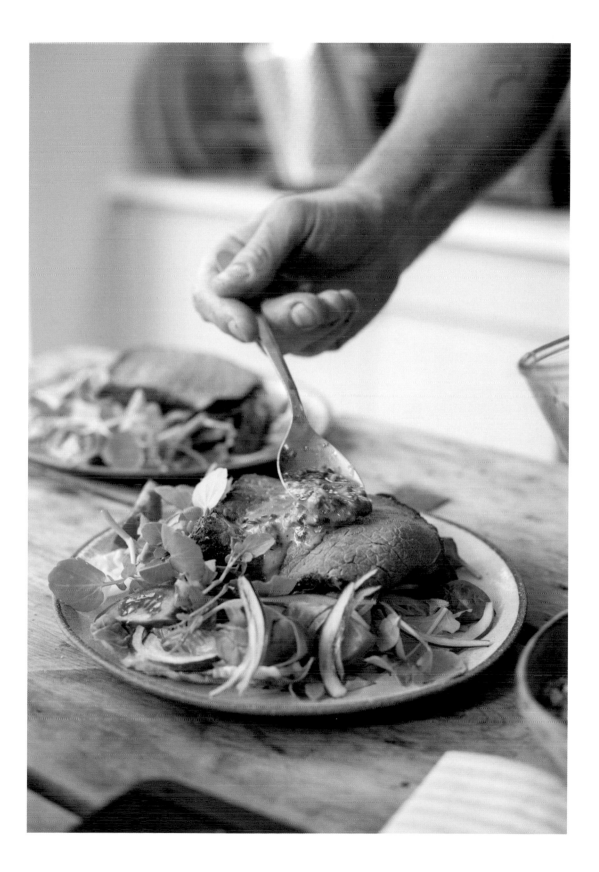

Chinese meatball stir-fry

The portion size here is massive: meaty mushrooms, loads of veg and four huge meatballs each – to satisfy the heartiest of appetites. Frying the meatballs first gives them a crispy, caramelised taste and texture on the outside, while they stay deliciously juicy inside. And the Asian flavours take the dish to another level.

Serves: 4

Calories: 445 per serving

1 tsp vegetable oil
2 onions, very finely chopped
1 tbsp light soy sauce
750g lean beef mince (5% fat)
1½ tsp Chinese five-spice powder
1½ tsp bicarbonate of soda
Sunflower oil spray
1 tsp sesame oil
1 large red onion, cut into
    thin wedges
200g carrots, thinly sliced on
    an angle
3 garlic cloves, finely chopped
2.5cm piece of ginger, finely grated
1 large red pepper, cored,
    deseeded and diced
1 large yellow pepper, cored,
    deseeded and diced
300ml fresh beef stock
120g mixed Asian mushrooms
    (such as oyster, shemeji and
    shiitake), sliced
1½ tbsp hoisin sauce
1½ tbsp oyster sauce
1 tbsp rice wine vinegar
1 tbsp cornflour
80g mangetout
4 spring onions, thinly sliced on
    an angle
Sea salt and freshly ground
    black pepper

1. Heat the vegetable oil in a non-stick frying pan over a medium heat. Add the chopped onions and cook for 5 minutes or until softened. Remove the pan from the heat and add the soy sauce. Leave to cool and allow the onions to soak up the soy.

2. Put the beef mince into a large bowl and add the cooled onions, Chinese five-spice, bicarbonate of soda and a good pinch each of salt and pepper. Mix well with your hands for 2–3 minutes. Divide the mixture into 16 equal pieces and roll into balls. Chill in the fridge for 2 hours to firm up.

3. Preheat the oven to fan 180°C/gas 4.

4. Place a large non-stick wok over a high heat. When it is hot, add 5–10 sprays of oil. Add the meatballs and cook for 5–6 minutes, or until browned on all sides. Transfer to an oven tray and cook in the oven for 10 minutes.

5. Meanwhile, return the wok to a high heat. Add the sesame oil, red onion and carrots and cook for 2 minutes. Toss in the garlic and ginger and cook for 2 minutes. Now add the red and yellow peppers and cook for 4 minutes. If the stir-fry begins to stick, add a dash of the beef stock to the pan to loosen.

6. Add the mushrooms, meatballs and half of the beef stock to the wok, then add the hoisin and oyster sauces and the rice wine vinegar. Stir well and bring to a simmer.

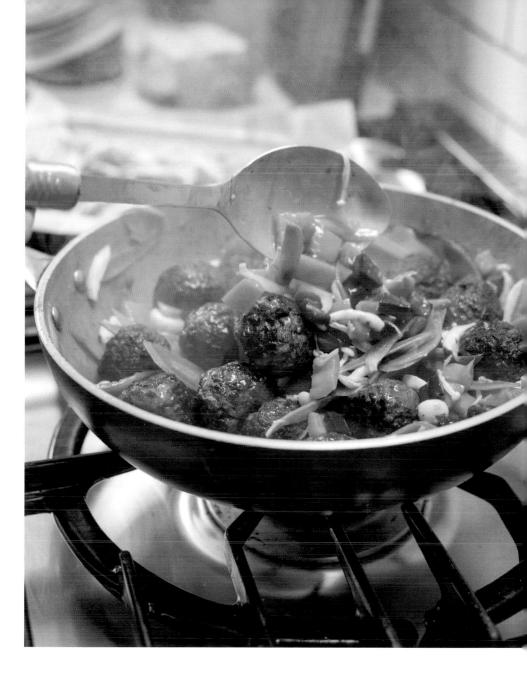

7. Mix the cornflour to a paste with 1 tbsp of the remaining beef stock and pour into the pan, along with the rest of the stock.

8. Add the mangetout and spring onions and stir-fry for 4–5 minutes or until the mangetout are just cooked and the meatballs are heated through. Divide between warmed bowls and serve.

Chilli con carne

This tasty, rich chilli has just a little melted cheese on top to give it a touch of indulgence and the tortilla adds a great crunchy texture. If you are looking for a lower calorie option though, you can leave out the tortillas.

Serves: 4

Calories: 720 per serving
480 without tortilla chips

1kg lean beef mince (5% fat)
2 tbsp cumin seeds
1 tbsp coriander seeds
1 tbsp vegetable oil
2 onions, diced
4 garlic cloves, finely chopped
1 tbsp paprika
½ tsp dried chilli flakes
1 tsp flaky sea salt
½ tsp freshly ground black pepper
500ml fresh beef stock
400g tin chopped tomatoes
2 tbsp tomato purée
300ml water

For the tortilla chips (optional)
4 medium corn tortillas, each cut
    into 8 wedges
Sunflower oil spray

To finish
80g mixture of grated half-fat
    Cheddar and half-fat mozzarella
40g pickled jalapeño chillies
A small handful of coriander leaves
Pickled pink onions (see page 172),
    optional

1. Preheat the oven to fan 180°C/gas 4.

2. Spread the beef out on a baking tray lined with baking parchment. Cook on the top shelf of the oven for 40 minutes, breaking up the mince well with a wooden spoon every 10 minutes. It should have a dark, even colour and resemble large coffee granules. Remove from the oven and set aside.

3. Meanwhile, toast the cumin seeds and coriander seeds in a small, dry pan until fragrant. Grind to a powder, using a coffee grinder or pestle and mortar.

4. Once the mince is cooked, heat the oil in a large non-stick sauté pan over a high heat. Add the diced onions and cook for 5 minutes to soften, adding a splash of water if they start to stick. Add the garlic and cook for a further 2 minutes, then lower the heat to medium.

5. Add the toasted ground spices, paprika, chilli, salt and pepper. Cook, stirring, for 1–2 minutes, then add the beef stock, tinned tomatoes, tomato purée and water to the pan. Bring to a simmer and add the browned beef mince. Simmer gently for 15–20 minutes until the sauce has thickened.

6. Meanwhile, for the tortilla chips if you're making them, lay the tortilla wedges on a large baking tray lined with baking parchment and spray with a few sprays of oil. Place the tray on the middle shelf of the oven and toast for 5–10 minutes or until the tortilla chips are brown and crispy.

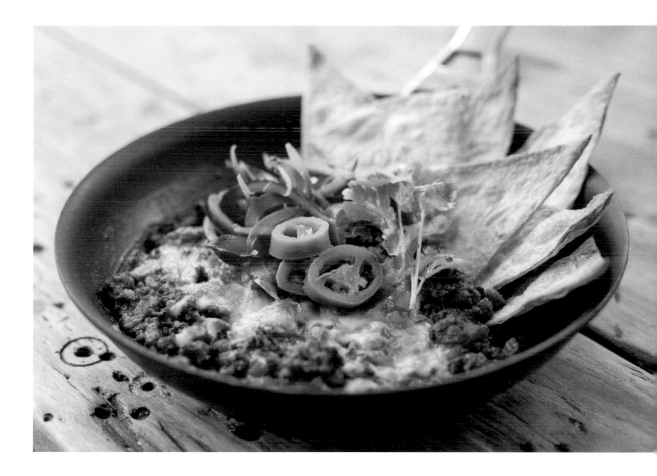

7. Transfer the chilli to an ovenproof dish and sprinkle the grated cheeses over the surface. Place on the top shelf of the oven for 10 minutes or until the cheese topping is melted and golden brown. Serve in warmed bowls, topped with the jalapeños and coriander. Finish with the pickled onions and tortilla chips, if serving.

....

THE LOWDOWN Thinking ahead is the key when you're dieting, so you're not tempted to resort to a takeaway or ready meal. This chilli can be made ahead and frozen. Defrost fully before reheating and finishing with the cheesy topping.

....

One-layer lasagne

This lighter version of the ever-popular pasta bake is layered with courgettes and beef tomatoes rather than pasta. The tasty ragu is made with lots of extra veg to boost the vitamins and minerals – and up the fibre content to keep you feeling full.

Serves: 6

Calories: 495 per serving

800g lean beef mince (5% fat)
1 tbsp light olive oil
2 large onions, finely diced
4 garlic cloves, grated
2 carrots, finely diced
2 celery sticks, finely diced
1 tbsp caraway seeds
3 tbsp tomato purée
700ml fresh beef stock
400g tin chopped tomatoes
1 crumbly beef stock cube
1 tbsp dried oregano
2 sprigs of rosemary, leaves
    stripped and finely chopped
200g button mushrooms, halved
2 large courgettes, thinly sliced
    on an angle
2 beef tomatoes, cut into 12 slices
250g ricotta
1 ball of mozzarella (125g), grated
10g grated Parmesan
Sea salt and freshly ground
    black pepper

For the lettuce with citrus dressing
Finely grated zest and juice of
    1 lime, 1 lemon and ½ grapefruit
70ml water
1 tbsp granulated sweetener
1 tbsp white wine vinegar
1 tbsp cornflour, mixed to a paste
    with 1 tbsp water
2 tbsp finely chopped chives
1 iceberg lettuce, cut into 6 wedges

1. Preheat the oven to fan 180°C/gas 4.

2. Spread the beef out on a baking tray lined with baking parchment. Cook on the top shelf of the oven for 40 minutes, breaking up the mince well with a wooden spoon every 10 minutes. It should have a dark, even colour and resemble large coffee granules. Remove and set aside.

3. Heat the oil in a large non-stick sauté pan. Add the onions and cook over a medium heat for 10 minutes or until softened, adding a splash of water if they start to stick. Add the garlic and cook for 1 minute, then add the carrots and celery and cook for 5 minutes. Sprinkle in the caraway seeds and cook for 30 seconds, then stir through the tomato purée and cook for 1 minute.

4. Add the browned mince, beef stock and tinned tomatoes. Crumble in the stock cube and add the herbs and mushrooms. Bring to the boil, then lower the heat to a simmer and cook for 25–30 minutes or until the sauce has thickened to a rich ragu.

5. Pour the ragu into an ovenproof dish, about 23 x 33cm and 5cm deep. Layer the courgettes, then the tomatoes on top, seasoning each layer with salt and pepper. Season the ricotta with salt and pepper and dot it evenly over the tomatoes.

6. Scatter the grated mozzarella and Parmesan over the surface and bake at fan 180°C/gas 4 for 35 minutes or until the topping is golden brown.

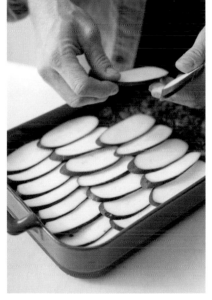

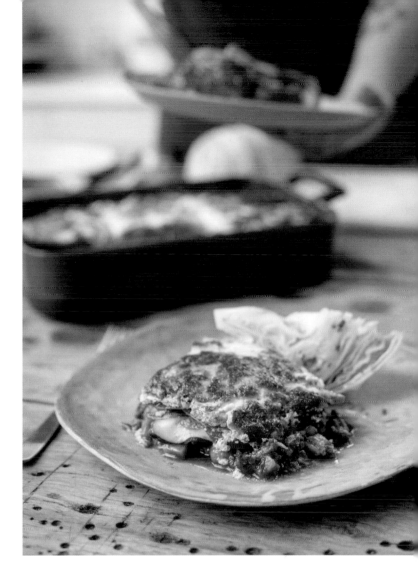

7. Meanwhile, for the salad dressing, put all the citrus zest and juice into a small saucepan with the water, sweetener and wine vinegar and bring up to a simmer over a medium heat. Take off the heat and whisk in the cornflour paste, then return to the heat and simmer, stirring, for 1–2 minutes until thickened a little. Leave to cool and then strain.

8. Stir the chopped chives into the cooled dressing and season with salt and pepper to taste.

9. Serve each portion of lasagne with a wedge of lettuce drizzled with some of the citrus dressing.

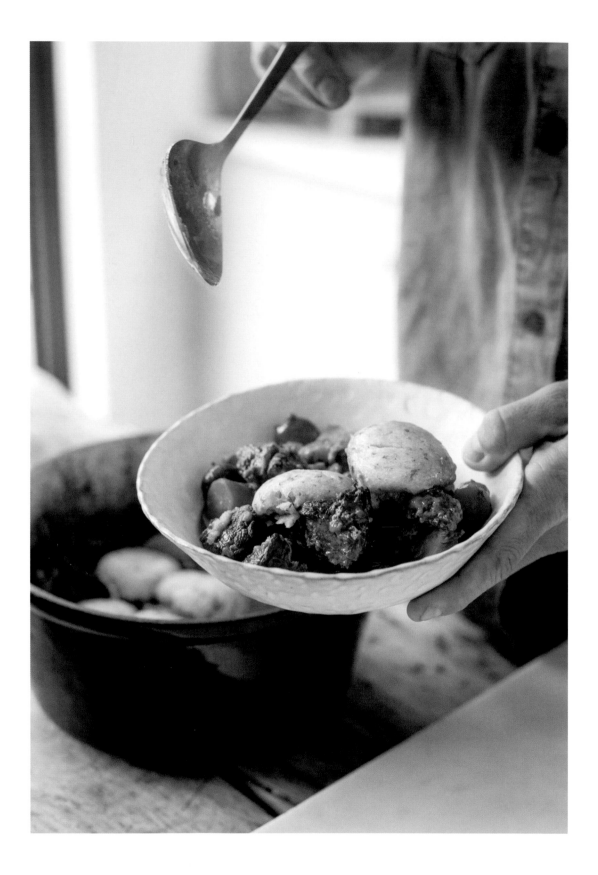

Beef stew and dumplings

Shin of beef is a flavoursome cut for stewing and you can trim off the fat. Try using other root veg here, such as swede, parsnips, celeriac or Jerusalem artichokes. The dumplings are made without suet, giving you the satisfaction with fewer calories.

Serves: 4

Calories: 530 per serving

1 tbsp vegetable oil
800g trimmed beef shin, cut into
    3cm chunks
1 large onion, finely diced
2 celery sticks, cut into
    3cm lengths
2cm piece of ginger, grated
500ml fresh beef stock
2 bay leaves
2 sprigs of rosemary
200g carrots, cut into 3cm chunks
300g baby turnips, peeled
    and halved
150g button mushrooms
2 tsp Dijon mustard
Sea salt and freshly ground
    black pepper
Chopped flat-leaf parsley, to finish

For the dumplings
100g self-raising flour
½ tsp flaky sea salt
25g butter
3 tbsp flat-leaf parsley leaves,
    finely chopped
50ml cold water

1. Preheat the oven to fan 150°C/gas 2.

2. Place a large non-stick, flameproof casserole over a high heat and add half the oil. When it is very hot, add half the beef with some salt and pepper and brown well on all sides, then transfer to a plate. Repeat with the rest of the beef. Set aside.

3. Add the onion to the casserole, lower the heat to medium and cook for 10 minutes until softened. If it begins to stick, add a splash of the stock. Add the celery and ginger and cook for 2–3 minutes.

4. Return the meat to the casserole and add the stock, bay leaves, rosemary and some salt and pepper. Bring to a simmer and put the lid on. Transfer to the oven and cook for 1¾ hours.

5. Take out the casserole and add the carrots, turnips and whole mushrooms. Stir, replace the lid and return to the oven for a further 45 minutes.

6. Meanwhile, for the dumplings, put the flour and salt into a bowl, rub in the butter with your fingertips and stir though the parsley and water. Gather the mix together to form a rough dough and divide into 8 pieces. Roll each into a ball and flatten slightly.

7. Take the casserole out of the oven, stir in the mustard and nestle the dumplings into the stew so they are half submerged in the liquor. Pop the lid back on and return to the oven for 20–30 minutes until the dumplings are cooked through. Serve in warmed bowls, scattered with a little extra parsley.

Pot-roast topside of beef

You can't beat a classic Sunday roast but it's so easy to eat almost your entire day's calories loaded onto one tasty plate! This pot roast has fewer calories but even more flavour and texture.

Serves: 6

Calories: 380 per serving

1.2kg joint of lean topside of beef,
    rolled and tied
1 tbsp olive oil
4 large onions, cut into wedges,
    leaving the root end intact
6 garlic cloves, sliced
2 tsp sweet smoked paprika
2 tbsp tomato purée
100ml red wine vinegar
600ml tinned beef consommé
A bunch of thyme (tied with string)
500g carrots, cut into roughly
    4cm lengths
8 celery sticks (350g in total),
    cut into roughly 4cm lengths
1 tbsp cornflour, mixed to a paste
    with 1 tbsp water
2 tbsp flat-leaf parsley leaves,
    finely chopped
Sea salt and freshly cracked
    black pepper

For the kale
100ml water
2 garlic cloves, grated
2 salted anchovies, finely chopped
150g kale, shredded
1 tbsp baby capers, roughly
    chopped
Finely grated zest of 1 lemon

1. Preheat the oven to fan 150°C/gas 2.

2. Dry the beef well with kitchen paper, then use a cook's blowtorch to sear the beef all over.

3. Heat the olive oil in a large non-stick flameproof casserole. Add the onions and fry for 10 minutes or until browned, adding a splash of water if they start to stick. Add the garlic, smoked paprika and tomato purée and cook for 2 minutes.

4. Pour in the wine vinegar, stir well, then pour in the beef consommé. Add the browned beef, thyme and carrots and bring to a simmer. Take off the heat and season with some salt and cracked pepper. Pop the lid on and cook in the oven for 2 hours.

5. Take the casserole out of the oven and turn the beef over. Add the celery and stir well. Return to the oven for 1½ hours or until the beef is tender.

6. At the end of the beef cooking time, cook the kale. Place a large non-stick sauté pan over a medium heat and add the 100ml water, garlic and anchovies. Cook for 2 minutes, then add the kale and cook for 4–5 minutes or until it wilts. Drain off excess water then stir through the capers and lemon zest. Season with pepper to taste.

7. Meanwhile, remove the casserole from the oven, lift out the beef joint and place it on a board to rest. Place the casserole over a medium heat, stir in the cornflour paste and cook, stirring, for 3–4 minutes or until the sauce is thickened slightly.

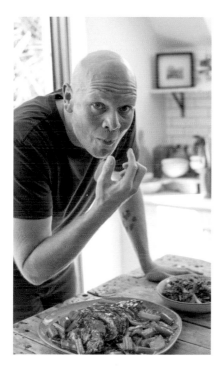

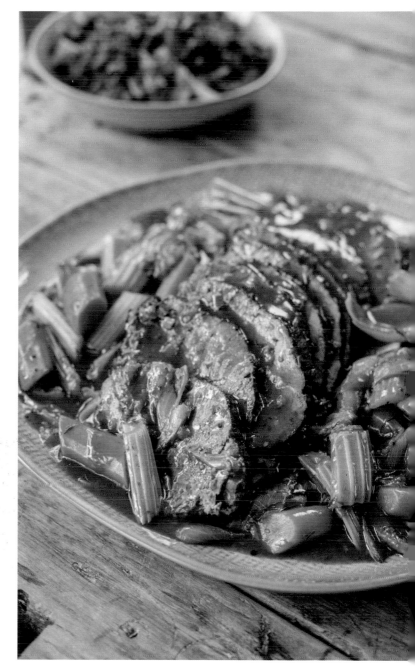

THE LOWDOWN Pot-roasting a joint of meat – on a bed of root veg in a covered pan with herbs – is a fantastic way to cook meat in its own juices, to retain all the flavour.

8. Cut the rested beef into thick slices and arrange on a platter with the veg from the casserole. Stir the chopped parsley through the sauce and spoon some over the beef slices. Serve with the rest of the sauce in a jug and the kale on the side.

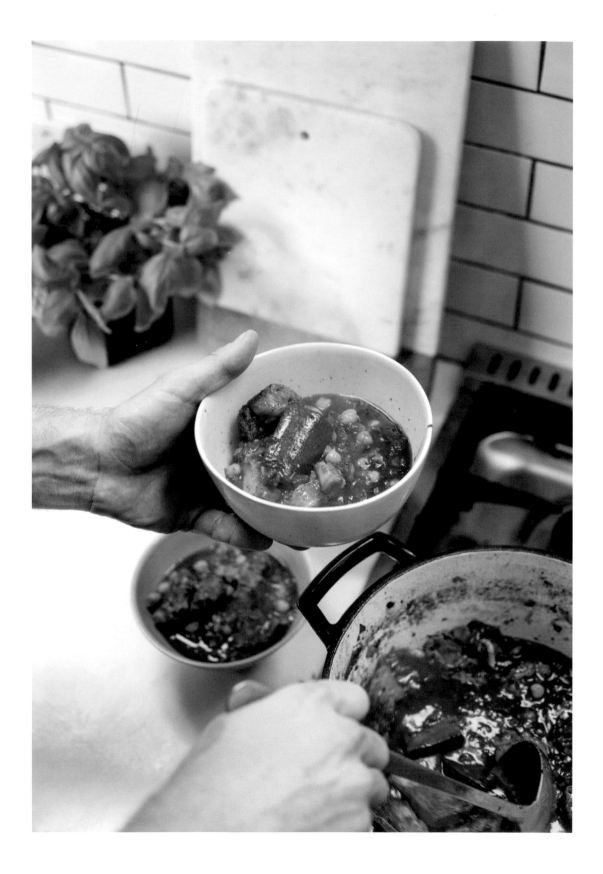

Lamb tagine with chickpeas

Lamb neck fillet is an excellent cut for slow cooking and braising and is slightly leaner than shoulder, which is more often used. Lamb stands up well to strong flavours like the harissa and dried mint in this aromatic tagine. There's also plenty of filling veg, like chickpeas and aubergine, making this a really sustaining meal.

Serves: 4

Calories: 590 per serving

800g lamb neck fillet, cut into
    5cm chunks
Sunflower oil spray
1 tbsp light olive oil
2 onions, diced
4 garlic cloves, finely diced
5cm piece of ginger, finely grated
1 tbsp rose harissa paste
    (without any oil)
2 tsp dried mint
1 cinnamon stick
500ml fresh lamb stock
400g tin chopped tomatoes
250g courgettes, cut into
    5cm long wedges
250g aubergine, cut into
    5cm long wedges
400g tin chickpeas
    (240g drained weight)
Sea salt and freshly ground
    black pepper
Coriander, roughly chopped,
    to finish

1. Preheat the oven to fan 160°C/gas 3.

2. Spray the lamb pieces on both sides with a little oil and season well with salt and pepper.

3. Heat a large flameproof casserole over a high heat on the hob. Brown the lamb (with no added oil) in batches on each side, then transfer to a plate.

4. Lower the heat under the casserole and add the olive oil. Toss in the onions and cook for 5 minutes or until softened. Add the garlic, ginger and harissa paste and cook for a further 2 minutes.

5. Add the dried mint, cinnamon, lamb stock, tomatoes and browned lamb and bring to a gentle simmer. Pop the lid on the casserole and cook in the oven for 1 hour.

6. Add the courgettes, aubergine and chickpeas to the casserole, stir well and put the lid back on. Return to the oven for a further 1 hour.

7. Remove from the oven and stir through some chopped coriander. Ladle into warmed bowls to serve.

Spicy lamb mince curry

There are definitely no subtle flavours going on here! This is all about big bold combinations and plenty of fiery spices. Puy lentils and finely chopped cauliflower give the curry plenty of body, so you won't necessarily need to serve rice on the side.

Serves: 4
Calories: 755 per serving 540 without rice

500g lean lamb mince (20% fat)
1 tbsp vegetable oil
2 onions, finely diced
6 garlic cloves, finely chopped
5cm piece of ginger, finely grated
1 or 2 long green chillies
   (depending how hot you like it),
   finely chopped
1 tbsp cumin seeds
1 tsp ground turmeric
1 tsp ground coriander
1 tbsp garam masala
1 tsp flaky sea salt
1 litre fresh lamb stock
250g packet pre-cooked
   Puy lentils
250g cauliflower florets,
   finely chopped
200g frozen peas
A handful of mint leaves, finely
   chopped
A handful of coriander leaves,
   finely chopped

To serve (optional)
240g basmati rice cooked with
   salt and a pinch of saffron
   strands

1. Preheat the oven to fan 180°C/gas 4.

2. Spread the minced lamb out on a baking tray lined with baking parchment and cook on the top shelf of the oven for 40 minutes, breaking it up well with a wooden spoon every 10 minutes. It should have a dark, even colour and resemble large coffee granules. Remove from the oven and set aside.

3. Heat the oil in a large non-stick sauté pan over a high heat. Add the onions and sauté for 5–6 minutes or until they are beginning to brown. Toss in the garlic, ginger and chilli(es) and cook, stirring, for 2 minutes.

4. Reduce the heat a little and add the spices and salt. Cook, stirring, for 1 minute then add the lamb stock and lentils. Increase the heat and bring to the boil then turn the heat down again and simmer for 5 minutes. Add the browned lamb mince and simmer for about 20 minutes, until the sauce has reduced and thickened slightly.

5. Add the cauliflower and cook for 10 minutes, then add the peas and cook for another 2 minutes. Remove from the heat and stir in the chopped mint and coriander. Serve the curry with the saffron rice, if you like.

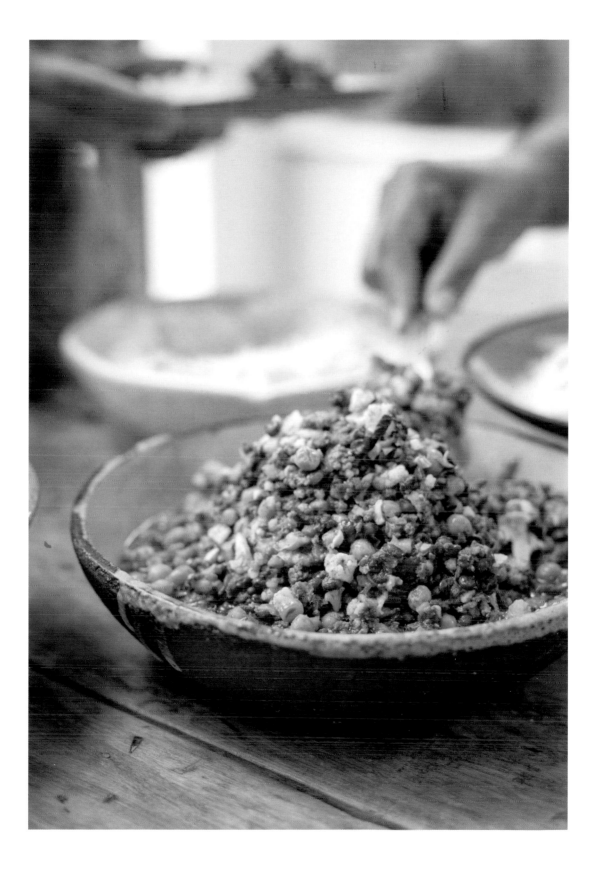

Lamb doner

Everyone is familiar with the favourite British late-night takeaway, but a typical doner kebab can be very high in calories. In this lower cal version, the spices are worked deep into the tender lamb leg meat and lamb mince by blitzing them together for a mouth-watering Middle Eastern blend.

Serves: 2

Calories: 650 per serving

For the lamb doner
175g lean lamb mince (20% fat)
175g lamb leg meat, trimmed of all fat
2 garlic cloves, finely grated
½ tsp flaky sea salt
½ tsp bicarbonate of soda
2 tsp ground cumin
1 tsp paprika
1 tsp onion powder
1 tsp dried oregano
A pinch of dried chilli flakes
Freshly ground black pepper

For the yoghurt sauce
100ml natural yoghurt (0% fat)
2 tbsp mint leaves, finely chopped
A pinch of granulated sweetener
A pinch of salt

To serve
2 medium corn tortillas
40g iceberg lettuce, shredded
50g cucumber, thinly sliced
2 tomatoes, sliced
½ small red onion, thinly sliced
6 pickled chillies
Hot sauce (optional)

1. Preheat the oven to fan 220°C/gas 7.

2. Place all the lamb doner ingredients in a food processor, adding plenty of pepper, and pulse until smooth. Divide the mixture in half. Shape each portion into a ball and roll out between two large sheets of greaseproof paper, until very thin.

3. Remove the top sheet of paper from each piece of meat. Place each rolled-out portion of meat, still on the bottom piece of paper, on a large oven tray. Place the trays on the top two shelves of the oven and cook for 3–4 minutes until browned.

4. Meanwhile, mix together all the ingredients for the yoghurt sauce.

5. Remove the trays from the oven and wave a cook's blowtorch all over the surface of the lamb until blackened in small areas. Leave to rest for a couple of minutes.

6. Warm the tortillas on the top shelf of the oven for a minute or so – or use a griddle pan. Place on warmed plates.

7. Slice the lamb into strips, about 2.5cm wide. Serve on the open tortillas with the salad, pickled chillies, a drizzle of the yoghurt dressing and maybe some hot sauce. These are generously filled tortillas, intended to be eaten open and not wrapped.

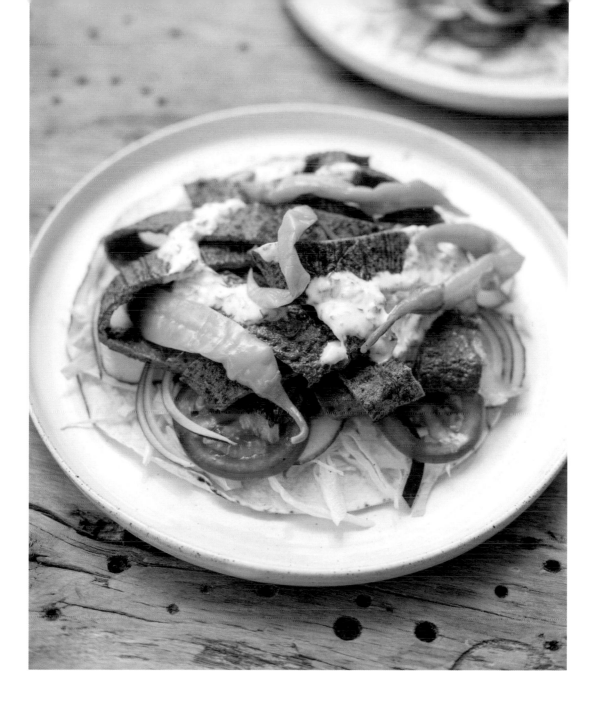

THE LOWDOWN Blowtorching the lamb after cooking it in the oven adds a great flavour to the meat, as well as crispness and an authentic chargrilled look.

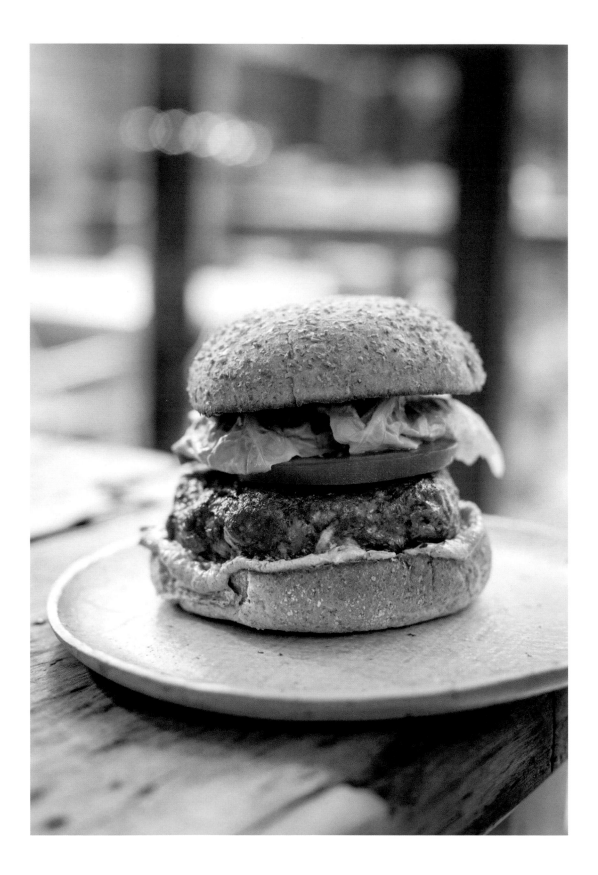

Spicy Moroccan lamb burgers

I love this Moroccan-spiced version of a classic lamb burger. Instead of the usual tzatziki topping, it uses a harissa-laced fat-free yoghurt sauce – which has a great combination of hot and cool tastes.

Serves: 4

Calories: 640 per serving
425 without bun

For the lamb burgers
1 large courgette, grated
100g peeled and grated carrot
    (about 1 large)
500g lean lamb mince (20% fat)
1 tsp bicarbonate of soda
1 large free-range egg,
    lightly beaten
30g fresh breadcrumbs
1 tbsp English mustard
1 tsp ground cinnamon
1 tbsp ras el hanout
1 tsp salt
1 tsp ground cumin
2 tsp dried mint
Freshly ground black pepper
Sunflower oil spray

For the harissa yoghurt
6 tbsp Greek yoghurt (0% fat)
2 tsp rose harissa paste

To serve
4 large wholemeal burger buns
1 large tomato, thickly sliced
2 little gem lettuce, leaves
    separated

1. Squeeze out any extra moisture from the grated courgette and carrot, then place in a bowl with all the other burger ingredients (apart from the spray oil), adding a generous grinding of pepper. Mix together thoroughly.

2. Divide the mixture into 4 portions and shape into large, fairly thin burger patties. Chill in the fridge for at least 2 hours, or overnight.

3. When you're ready to cook your burgers, mix together the yoghurt and harissa and set aside. Halve and toast the wholemeal burger buns.

4. Preheat the grill to high. Spray a baking tray a few times with oil and place the burgers on the tray. Spray the top of each burger a few times with oil. Cook under the hot grill for 5–6 minutes on each side, until nicely browned.

5. Spread the harissa yoghurt on the bottom of each burger bun, add a burger, then top with a tomato slice and some lettuce. Pop the lid on and tuck in.

Pork tenderloin with Japanese ponzu dressing

Pork fillet is a lovely lean cut of meat that works well with an intense marinade like this one. The pak choi goes brilliantly, and the dressing – with its citrusy yuzu, soy and mirin flavours and seaweed flakes – rounds off this fragrant light dish perfectly.

Serves: 2

Calories: 420 per serving

500g pork fillet, cut into 2 pieces
Sunflower oil spray
3 pak choi, halved lengthways
4 tbsp water
1 tsp sesame seeds, toasted

For the marinade
1 tbsp light soy sauce
1 tbsp Shaoxing wine
2 garlic cloves, crushed
2.5cm piece of ginger, finely grated

For the ponzu dressing
2 tbsp mirin
1 tbsp light soy sauce
½ tbsp rice wine vinegar
½ tbsp yuzu juice
½ tsp kombu seaweed flakes

. . . .

THE LOWDOWN This easy marinade adds instant flavour – try it with chicken breasts or thighs too.

. . . .

1. Put the marinade ingredients into a small ziplock bag and mix well. Add the pork and close the bag. Mix well and massage the marinade into the pork then leave to marinate in the fridge for 1 hour.

2. Meanwhile, make the ponzu dressing. Put all the ingredients into a small saucepan and bring to the boil, then lower the heat and simmer for 4 minutes. Leave to cool, then strain into a jug and pour into two dipping bowls.

3. When ready to cook the pork, preheat the oven to fan 180°C/gas 4. Line a baking tray with baking parchment. Take the pork out of the fridge.

4. Heat a non-stick frying pan over a very high heat. When hot, add 6–10 sprays of oil. Add the pork and cook for 2–3 minutes on each side or until it is an even, dark brown colour on all sides.

5. Transfer the pork to the lined tray and cook on the top shelf of the oven for 7 minutes. Remove and set aside to rest while you cook the pak choi.

6. Add the halved pak choi to the frying pan, cut side down, and sear over a medium-high heat. Add the 4 tbsp water and cook the pak choi for 2 minutes on each side.

7. Slice the pork fillet and sprinkle with toasted sesame seeds. Serve with the ponzu dipping sauce and pak choi.

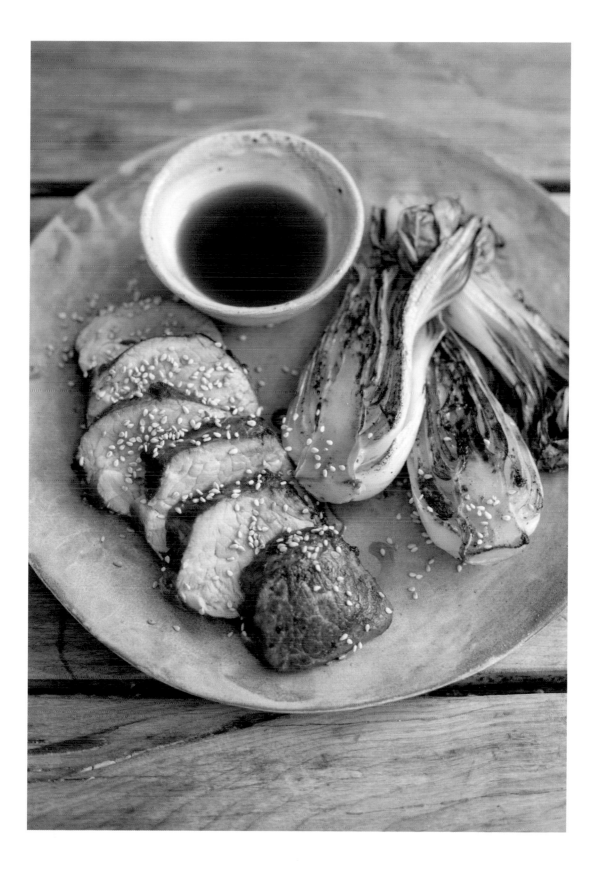

Pork samosa pie

Roasting the pork for this 'samosa pie' beforehand intensifies the taste and, once it is combined with all those amazing spices and the crunchy filo, it really is like eating a samosa – just a lighter version that hasn't been deep-fried.

Serves: 6

Calories: 475 per serving

1kg lean pork mince (5% fat)
1 tbsp light olive oil
2 large onions, finely diced
4 garlic cloves, finely chopped
4 long green chillies,
    finely chopped
1 tbsp cumin seeds
½ tsp ground cardamom
2 tbsp medium Madras curry
    powder
1 tsp flaky sea salt
400g tin beef consommé
400ml chicken stock
400g potatoes, peeled and diced
250g frozen peas
3 sheets of filo pastry
1 tsp nigella seeds

1. Preheat the oven to fan 180°C/gas 4. Line a deep, lipped baking tray with baking parchment.

2. Spread the mince out on the baking tray and cook on the top shelf of the oven for 40 minutes, breaking it up well with a wooden spoon every 10 minutes. It should have a dark, even colour and resemble large coffee granules. Remove and set aside. Lower the oven setting to fan 170°C/gas 3.

3. Heat the oil in a large non-stick sauté pan over a high heat. Add the onions and cook for 5 minutes or until softened, adding a splash of water if they start to stick. Add the garlic, chillies and cumin seeds and cook for a further 4 minutes; again add a splash of water if the mixture starts to stick.

4. Stir in the cardamom, curry powder and salt and cook, stirring, for 1 minute. Pour in the beef consommé and chicken stock, add the cooked pork mince and potatoes and bring to a simmer. Cook for 20 minutes, or until the potatoes are cooked and the sauce has thickened.

5. Stir the peas through the pork and potato mixture and transfer to a 30 x 25cm roasting tin.

6. Cut each filo sheet in half. Spray one piece 4 or 5 times with oil, then sprinkle with a few nigella seeds and scrunch it a bit. Lay the pastry, oiled-side up, over the pork. Repeat with the remaining pastry.

7. Bake the pie on the middle shelf of the oven for 20–25 minutes or until the filo is brown and crispy.

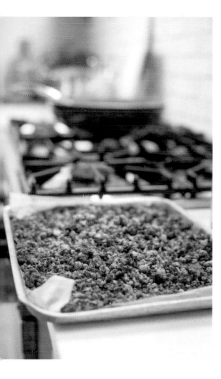

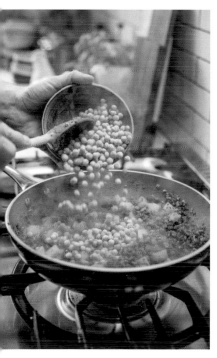

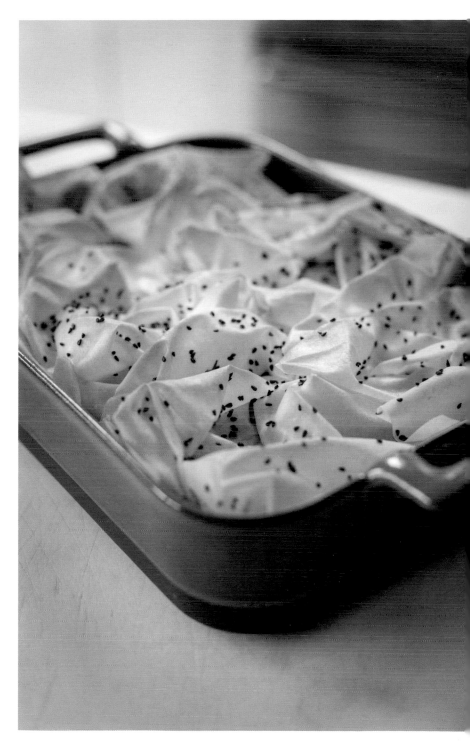

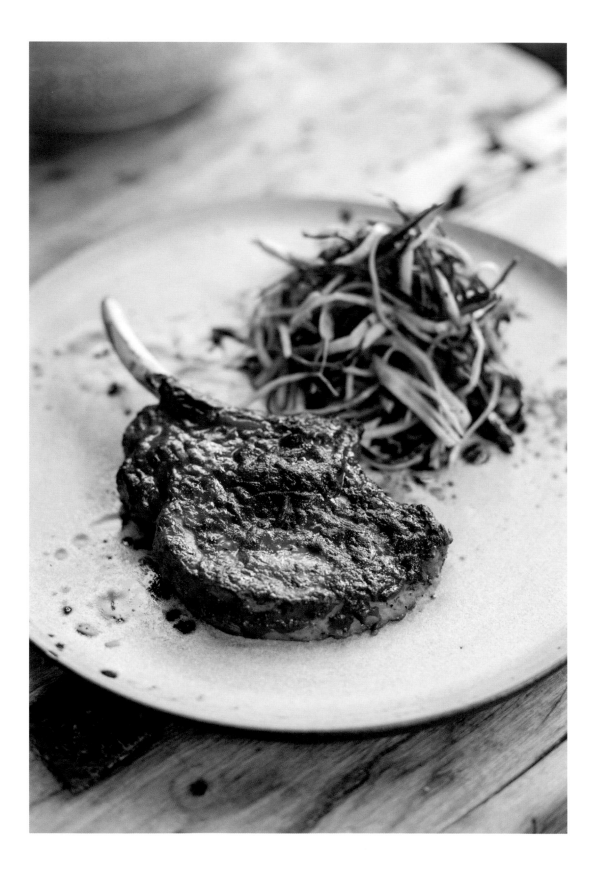

Sticky pork chops

This recipe taps into everyone's love of those all-American smoky flavours. It has a great barbecue-style glaze, but with much less added sugar. A fresh and crunchy slaw is the perfect foil for the sticky chops.

Serves: 2
Calories: 420 per serving

2 trimmed bone-in pork chops,
   i.e. all fat removed (250g each)
Olive oil spray
Sea salt and freshly ground
   black pepper

For the barbecue sauce
4 tbsp tomato ketchup
1 tbsp maple syrup
1 tbsp Worcestershire sauce
1 tbsp English mustard
½ tsp cayenne pepper

For the slaw
100g red cabbage, finely shredded
100g white cabbage, finely
   shredded
1 tbsp white wine vinegar
2 tbsp Greek yoghurt (0% fat)

1. Preheat the oven to fan 240°C/gas 9. Line an oven tray with baking parchment.

2. Season the pork chops on both sides with salt and pepper. Heat a griddle pan over a high heat. Spray both sides of the chops with a few sprays of oil. When the griddle is smoking hot, add the chops and cook for 2 minutes on each side or until well charred. Set aside on the lined oven tray.

3. For the barbecue sauce, mix all the ingredients together in a small bowl.

4. Coat the pork chops in the sauce, on both sides. Cook on the top shelf of the oven for 10 minutes or until cooked through.

5. Meanwhile, mix together all the ingredients for the slaw and season with salt and pepper.

6. Remove the pork chops from the oven and run a cook's blowtorch over them to blacken slightly. Serve with the crunchy slaw.

Pulled pork tacos

This meaty sharing dish is very easy to cook, as you let the oven do all the work. The secret is to cut the fat off the pork, then rub the meat with the marinade and leave it – overnight if possible – to take in all those amazing flavours. Slow cooking produces incredibly succulent, moist meat with that fantastic pull-apart tender texture. The tortilla cases and vibrant salad provide a lovely crunchy contrast.

Serves: 8

Calories: 450 per serving

1.8kg trimmed joint of boneless pork shoulder (i.e. fat removed)

For the marinade
100g chipotle paste
2 tbsp tomato purée
3 tbsp cider vinegar
Juice of 2 oranges
2 garlic cloves, grated
2 tsp dried oregano
1 tsp flaky salt
1 tsp ground nutmeg
1 tsp ground allspice
1 tsp hot smoked paprika
1 tsp ground cumin

For the pickled pink onions
2 red onions, thinly sliced
1 tsp flaky sea salt
½ tsp dried oregano
½ tsp cumin seeds, lightly crushed
2 tbsp cider vinegar
Juice of 1 lime

To serve
8 medium corn tortillas
Sunflower oil spray
1 iceberg lettuce, shredded
400g tomatoes, diced
2 handfuls of coriander leaves

1. Mix all the marinade ingredients together in a small bowl. Place the pork in a non-reactive bowl, add the marinade and turn to coat. Cover with cling film and leave to marinate in the fridge for at least a couple of hours, ideally overnight.

2. When ready to cook, preheat the oven to fan 140°C/gas 1. Place the pork and marinade in a roasting dish and cover tightly with foil, making sure it's well sealed. Cook on a low oven shelf for 4 hours.

3. Meanwhile, for the pickled onions, put the red onions into a small bowl, pour on 350ml boiling water and leave to stand for 10 minutes. Drain and return the onions to the bowl. Add the salt, oregano, cumin seeds, cider vinegar and lime juice. Mix well, then cover with cling film and place in the fridge for 2 hours. The onions will pickle and turn pink.

4. When the pork is cooked, remove from the oven and set aside, still covered, to rest for 20 minutes while you make the tacos.

5. Turn the oven up to fan 180°C/gas 4.

6. Take two muffin trays and turn them upside down. Lay a tortilla over each of two mounds on each tray and poke them down the sides to create two bowl shapes. Spray with 4–6 sprays of oil. Bake for 7–8 minutes or until the tortilla cases are golden brown. Repeat with the remaining tortillas.

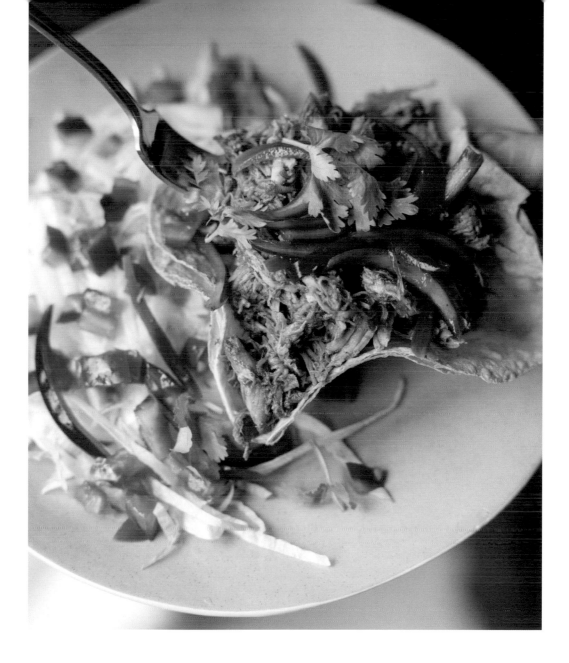

7. Remove the foil from the pork and shred the meat, using two forks. Mix the pork well with the marinade and pan juices. Place back in the oven for 15 minutes or so to heat up.

8. Place a tortilla bowl on each plate and fill with a pile of pulled pork. Arrange the shredded lettuce and tomatoes on the side. Top with the pickled pink onions and coriander then serve straight away.

Pea and ham pasta

The joy of this one is that it's so quick to make – just 20 minutes from start to finish! Anchovies and lemon zest work well together and you don't need much of them to add a really punchy flavour. Crème fraîche and Parmesan give the dish a touch of indulgence, while herbs add freshness at the end. A brilliant weekday meal.

Serves: 2

Calories: 585 per serving

175g lumaca rigate pasta (or
    other pasta shapes, see below)
1 tsp olive oil
1 large onion, diced
3 slices of Parma ham (45g in
    total), roughly torn
2 large garlic cloves, finely grated
4 salted anchovies, chopped
120g frozen peas
A handful of mint leaves,
    finely chopped
A handful of parsley leaves,
    finely chopped
20g grated Parmesan
60ml half-fat crème fraîche
Sea salt and freshly ground
    black pepper
Grated zest of ½ lemon, to finish

1. Cook the pasta in a large pan of boiling salted water until *al dente*. This will take about 10 minutes.

2. Meanwhile, heat the olive oil in a medium sauté pan over a medium heat and add the onion and Parma ham. Sweat for 3–4 minutes or until the onion has softened. Add the garlic and anchovies and cook for 2 minutes.

3. Add the peas to the pasta and then drain, reserving about a ladleful of the cooking water.

4. Add enough of the reserved pasta water to the onion and Parma ham mixture to loosen the sauce – you may not need it all – and stir well.

5. Add the herbs, Parmesan and crème fraîche then season with salt and pepper to taste.

6. Toss the pasta in the sauce to coat, spoon into warmed serving bowls and sprinkle with lemon zest to serve.

THE LOWDOWN *Lumaca rigate* literally means 'grooved snails'. This small shell-shaped pasta is great for holding thick sauces. If you can't get hold of it, use conchiglie, short macaroni, penne, rigatoni or fusilli instead.

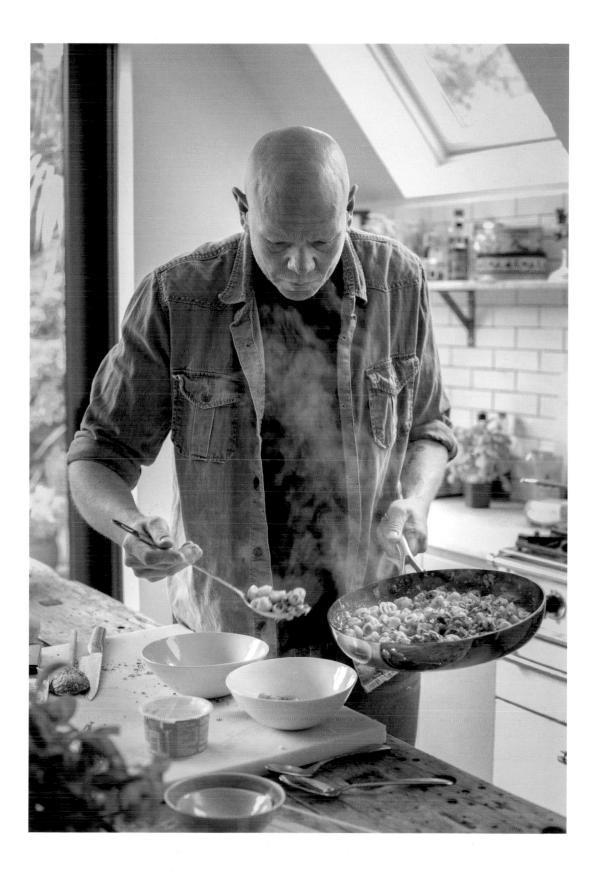

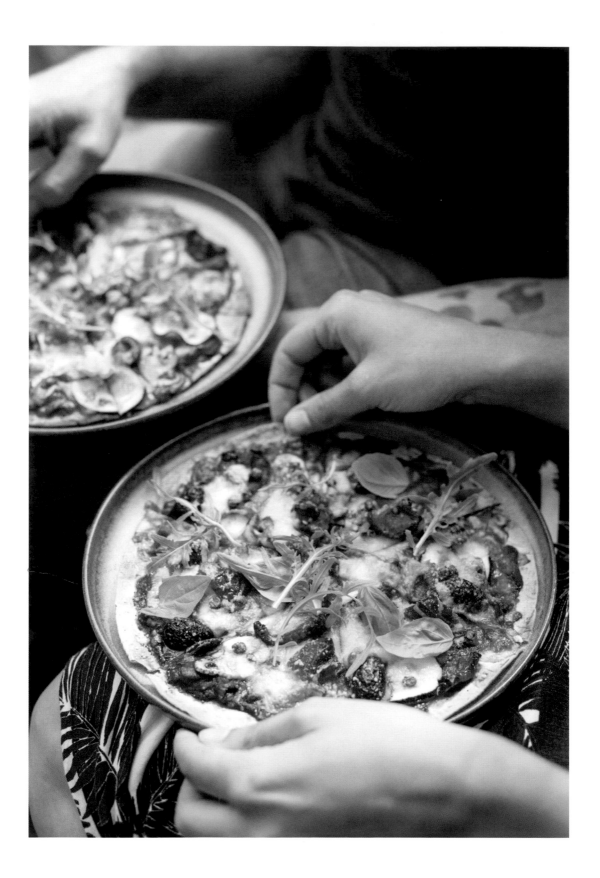

Easy pizza with Parma ham and mozzarella

Pizza is the perfect grab and share dinner but it's usually pretty high in calories, with a thick doughy crust and a hefty cheese topping. This version uses a healthy, thin tortilla base for a super tasty low-cal alternative, with a speedy tomato sauce and all your favourite toppings.

Serves: 2

Calories: 440 per pizza

2 large corn (or wheat) tortillas
180g tinned chopped tomatoes
1 tbsp tomato purée
2 sprigs of oregano, leaves picked
    and finely chopped
1 garlic clove, finely grated
Sea salt and freshly ground
    black pepper

For the topping
2 mushrooms, thinly sliced
12 thin slices of courgette
30g pitted black olives, halved
3 salted anchovies, finely chopped
2 tsp baby capers
6 sun-blushed tomatoes, halved
3 slices of Parma ham (45g in
    total), roughly torn
4 slices of reduced-fat salami
    (20g in total), halved
100g half-fat mozzarella, grated
10g grated Parmesan

To finish
Basil and rocket leaves

1. Preheat the oven to fan 150°C/gas 2.

2. Place the tortillas on two baking trays and bake for 5 minutes or until crispy but not coloured.

3. Meanwhile, mix together the tinned tomatoes, tomato purée, oregano and garlic. Add a pinch each of salt and pepper and stir well.

4. Remove the tortillas from the oven. Increase the setting to fan 180°C/gas 4.

5. Spread half of the tomato mixture evenly over each tortilla, leaving a 1cm clear margin all round. Divide the topping ingredients between the tortillas, finishing with the mozzarella and a final scattering of Parmesan.

6. Bake the pizzas in the oven for 10–12 minutes or until the cheese has melted and started to turn golden brown.

7. Cut the pizzas into wedges and scatter over the basil and rocket leaves to serve.

THE LOWDOWN You can make your own sun-blushed tomatoes: arrange tomato halves on a baking tray, season with salt and pepper, add a spray of oil and cook slowly at fan 55°C/lowest gas for about 6 hours.

VEGGIE

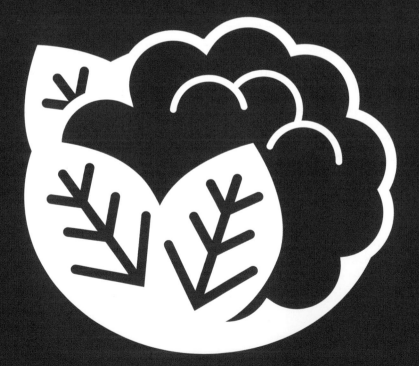

Introducing more vegetables to mealtimes is an easy way of cutting back on calories, while increasing fibre intake. Replacing just a few of your regular meat-based meals each week with veggie dishes will help you on your way to reaching your weight-loss goal.

Think of veg as more than just a supporting act on your plate. If you are a meat lover, chickpeas, beans, aubergine and mushrooms are great alternatives, as they are substantial and have a satisfying, hearty texture. They are also good at taking on the flavours of ingredients they are cooked with. The Chickpea and spinach curry (page 192) and Japanese miso aubergine (page 211) are fantastic, quick meals with interesting flavours that you can knock up in next to no time after work. And if you're really ravenous, Sweet potato and black bean burritos (page 204) is one of the most filling recipes in this book.

One of my favourite new additions to a diet-friendly kitchen is the spiralizer, which is really just a jazzed-up grater. Okay, so you may think I've gone a step too far here, but trust me, spiralizers are amazing! As a very low-calorie alternative to spaghetti, spiralized courgettes are brilliant – and they taste much better too. Try my 'courgetti' with homemade pesto on page 207 once, and you'll be making it every week.

Another new ingredient that I've come to love is cauliflower 'rice'. You can buy it ready-made in packets, but as with all things, it's better if you make your own. You can do this simply by grating raw cauliflower on a box grater, or blitzing it in a food processor. All that extra fibre will fill you up for virtually none of the calories of regular rice. I've used cauliflower rice in Stuffed peppers (page 196), and also in my Jerk chicken rice 'n' peas (page 116) and Chicken biryani (page 132). It means the portion sizes are *huge*, which is a real bonus when you're on a diet.

There are so many ways to enjoy vegetables – and there are so many amazing veg out there to try. I'm hoping these recipes will inspire you to get experimenting with them in the kitchen.

Pickled beetroot hummus with crudités

This easy-to-make hummus is such a lush and amazing colour and it's packed with flavour. You can serve it with loads of things – toasted pitta bread is great to scoop it up, or just some simple raw veg, like radish, celery, carrot, cucumber or fennel, to dip. Just be sure to buy the beetroot from the chilled salad section of the supermarket – the pickled beetroot you buy in a jar is too vinegary.

Serves: 4

Calories: 600 per serving
365 without pitta

500g cooked pickled beetroot
   (see above)
2 x 400g tins chickpeas
1 tbsp ground cumin, toasted
2 garlic cloves, finely grated
2 tbsp tahini
Juice of 2 lemons
A handful of mint leaves,
   roughly chopped
100g Greek yoghurt (0% fat)
Sea salt and freshly ground
   black pepper

To finish
80g half-fat feta
1 tbsp fennel seeds, toasted
A handful of small mint leaves

To serve
Raw veg (small peeled carrots,
   radishes, cherry tomatoes,
   cucumber batons, celery sticks,
   fennel slices)
4 wholemeal pittas, toasted
   (optional)

1. Put the beetroot into a food processor and blitz until smooth.

2. Drain the chickpeas, reserving the liquid. Add the chickpeas to the blender with 150ml of the liquid. Add the toasted cumin, garlic, tahini, lemon juice and mint. Blend again until smooth.

3. Season generously with salt and pepper, add the yoghurt and blitz again until smooth.

4. Transfer the hummus to a serving bowl, crumble over the feta and sprinkle with the toasted fennel seeds and mint leaves. Serve with the raw veg crudités for dipping and toasted pitta, if you like.

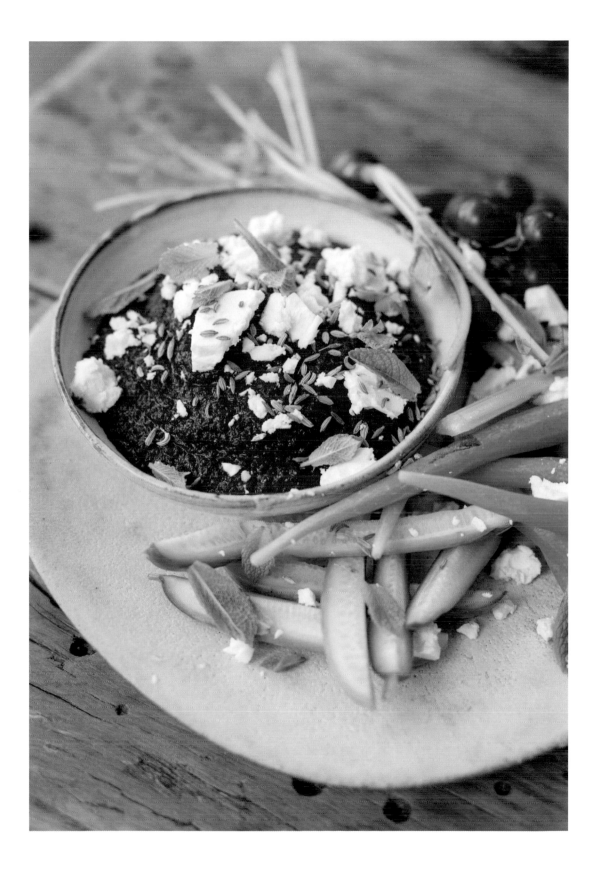

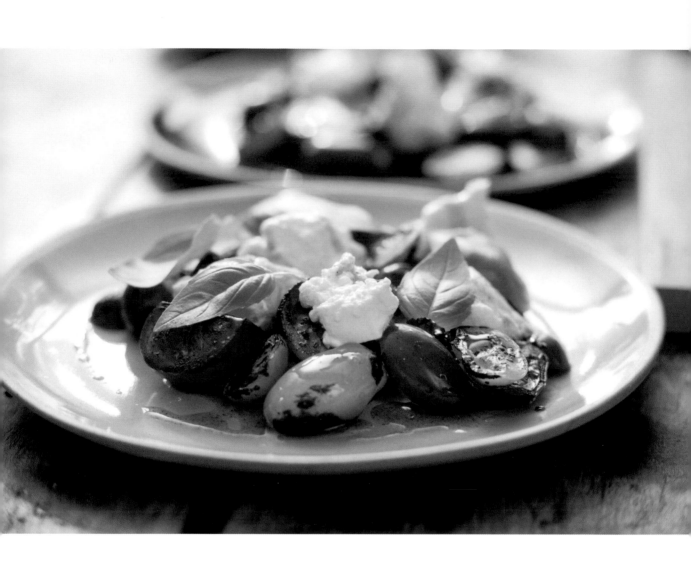

THE LOWDOWN Blowtorching the tomatoes may sound fancy but it's an easy way to fire-roast them for an amazing smoky taste – browning the skins without cooking the flesh.

Tomato, ricotta and basil salad

This colourful salad is a low-calorie version of the Italian favourite, *tricolore*, which normally uses mozzarella. I've swapped it for naturally lower fat ricotta, and a clever oil-free paprika dressing brings it all together. You will have more dressing than you need for this recipe, so keep the rest in the fridge (for up to a week) to use whenever you need a low-fat flavour boost.

Serves: 2

Calories: 150 per serving

400g heritage tomatoes (a mix of larger and cherry tomatoes, ideally including red and yellow varieties)
100g ricotta
A small handful of basil leaves, larger leaves torn
Sea salt and freshly ground black pepper

For the smoked paprika dressing
220ml water
2 tbsp white wine vinegar
1 heaped tsp sweet smoked paprika
1 tbsp granulated sweetener
½ tsp garlic powder
½ tsp dried herbes de Provence
1 tsp salt
1 tbsp cornflour, mixed to a paste with 1 tbsp water

1. First make the dressing. Put the water, wine vinegar, smoked paprika, sweetener, garlic powder, dried herbs and salt into a small pan and bring to a simmer. Take off the heat and whisk in the cornflour paste. Return to the heat and cook for 1–2 minutes or until slightly thickened. Leave to cool completely, then strain into a jug.

2. Quarter the large tomatoes and halve the cherry tomatoes. Spread them all out, skin side up, on a metal tray and wave a cook's blowtorch over the surface until the skins are charred and blistered in places, then turn the tomatoes and colour the cut surfaces.

3. Arrange the tomatoes on individual plates and season with salt and pepper to taste. Dollop the ricotta on top and scatter over the basil leaves. Drizzle with 3 tbsp of the smoked paprika dressing to serve.

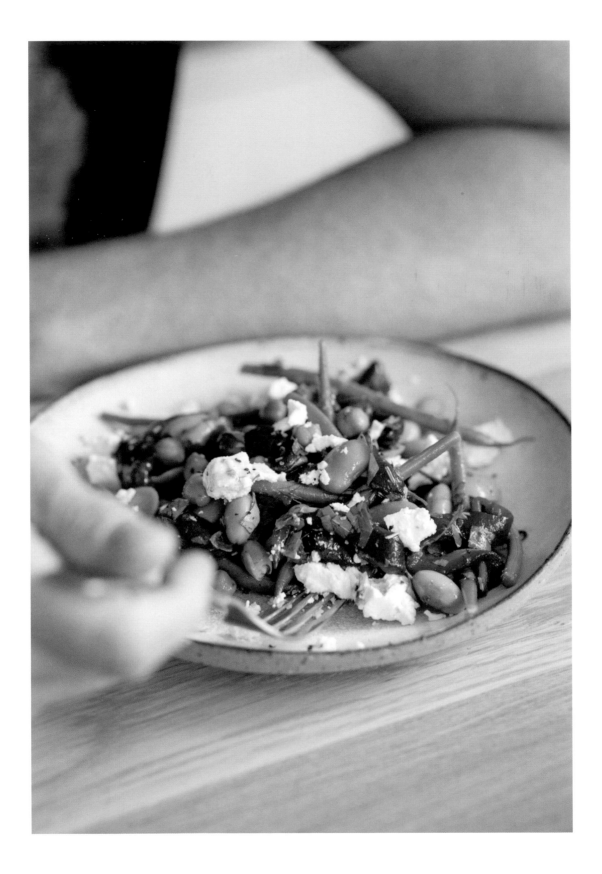

Mixed bean, roasted pepper and feta salad

This makes a great light lunch, or you can serve a smaller portion as a side dish with some simply cooked chicken, lamb or fish. It has a really nice, sharp dressing that you can use for other salads and veg dishes – a little goes a long way.

Serves: 4

Calories: 345 per serving

4 large red peppers
Olive oil spray
150g fine green beans
2 x 400g tins mixed beans,
    rinsed and drained
80g pitted green olives
2 handfuls of flat-leaf parsley
    leaves, roughly chopped
A handful of basil leaves,
    roughly chopped
120g half-fat feta
Freshly ground black pepper

For the dressing
2 tbsp extra virgin olive oil
3 tbsp red wine vinegar
1 small garlic clove, finely grated
1 tsp dried rosemary
1 tsp flaky sea salt
½ tsp freshly ground black pepper

1. Preheat the oven to fan 240°C/gas 9.

2. Place the red peppers in a small roasting tray and spray each one twice with oil. Roast on the top shelf of the oven for 15–20 minutes, or until well charred on all sides.

3. Transfer the roasted peppers to a bowl, cover with cling film and leave for 20 minutes to cool down; the trapped steam will help loosen the skins.

4. Meanwhile, add the green beans to a pan of boiling salted water and blanch them for a couple of minutes until cooked but still firm to the bite. Drain and place in a bowl of cold water to cool, then drain well.

5. Peel away the skin from the cooled peppers, remove the core and seeds then cut the flesh into long, thick slices. Place these in a bowl and add the green beans, tinned beans, olives, parsley and basil. Toss lightly to mix.

6. For the dressing, whisk all the ingredients together in a bowl. Pour over the salad, mix well and leave to stand for a few minutes to allow the salad to soak up the dressing.

7. Divide the salad between four plates, crumble over the feta and grind over some black pepper.

Griddled veg and halloumi with couscous

Griddled halloumi has a lovely, salty tang so you don't need much to make an impact in this Mediterranean salad. The herb dressing is a great recipe to have in your arsenal – it has a satisfying consistency with virtually no calories. You will have more than you need, so keep the rest in the fridge (for up to a week) to add instant flavour to veg and other salads.

Serves: 4 as a main, 6 as a side

**Calories: 440 per serving as a main
295 as a side or mezze dish**

150g couscous
150ml hot fresh vegetable stock
1 each red, yellow and green
    pepper, cored, deseeded and
    cut into 2cm slices
1 large red onion, cut into wedges
1 medium courgette, sliced
    into thick rounds
Olive oil spray
250g block of halloumi
Sea salt and freshly ground
    black pepper

For the herb dressing
200ml water
2 tbsp red wine vinegar
1 tsp garlic powder
½ tsp dried herbes de Provence
½ tsp dried Italian herb mix
1 tsp granulated sweetener
1 tsp flaky sea salt
1 tbsp cornflour, mixed to a paste
    with 1 tbsp water
2 tbsp flat-leaf parsley leaves,
    finely chopped

To finish (optional)
Basil and mint leaves
**1 red chilli, deseeded and sliced
    on an angle**

1. Put the couscous into a small bowl, add a pinch each of salt and pepper and pour on the hot veg stock. Stir well, cover with cling film and set aside.

2. For the herb dressing, put the water, wine vinegar, garlic powder, dried herbs, sweetener and salt into a small pan and bring to a simmer. Take off the heat, whisk in the cornflour paste, then return to the heat and cook for 1–2 minutes until slightly thickened. Pour into a jug and leave to cool, then stir in the chopped parsley.

3. Place all the veg in a large bowl and season with salt and pepper. Heat a large griddle pan over a high heat, then spray with about 20 sprays of oil. Lay about half the veg in the pan, being careful not to overcrowd it, and spray them with another 20 sprays of oil. Cook for 4–5 minutes on each side, until just softened and with some char lines, then remove to a plate. Repeat with the remaining veg.

4. Cut the halloumi in half lengthways and then cut each half into 6 slices. Spray the griddle pan again with oil and lay the halloumi slices in the pan. Cook over a high heat for 2 minutes on each side.

5. Fluff up the couscous with a fork and spoon onto a large platter. Top with the roasted veg and halloumi, then tear over the basil and mint leaves and scatter over the chilli, if using. Drizzle 6 tbsp of the herb dressing over everything and serve.

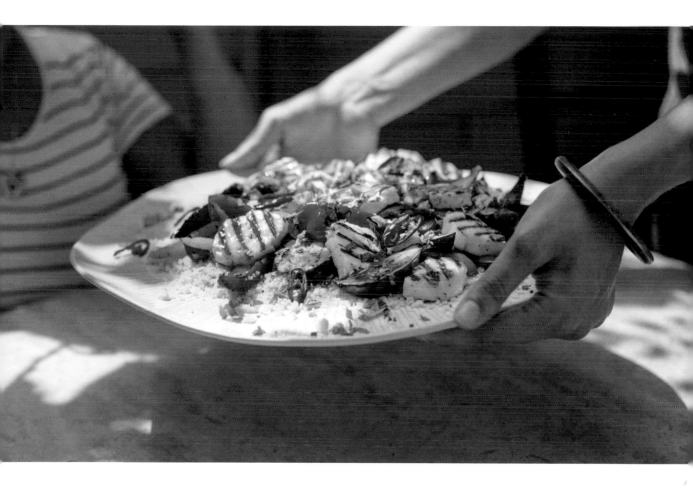

Spiced red salad

This vibrant, crunchy salad goes with virtually anything. It's really tasty too – perfect for when you need an interesting veggie side dish.

Serves: 4

Calories: 210 per serving

300g red cabbage, finely shredded
1 large red onion, finely sliced
1 tbsp flaky sea salt
2 oranges
2 red apples, julienned (skin on)
200g cooked beetroot
   (not in vinegar), julienned
150g fennel, finely sliced,
   fronds reserved
30g pecan nuts, toasted and
   chopped
A handful of dill leaves

For the dressing
½ tbsp wholegrain mustard
Finely grated zest and juice of
   1 orange
1 tbsp extra virgin olive oil
2 tbsp red wine vinegar

1. Put the cabbage and onion into a bowl, sprinkle with the flaky salt and mix well. Leave to stand for 20 minutes.

2. Meanwhile, segment the oranges: trim off the top and bottom and stand the fruit on a board. Work your way around each orange with a small, sharp knife, cutting off the peel, pith and outer membrane. Then, over a large bowl to catch the juice, slice between the membranes to release the orange segments into the bowl.

3. Rinse the shredded cabbage and onion in a sieve under cold running water to remove the salt, and drain well.

4. Add the cabbage and onion, apples, beetroot, fennel and pecans to the orange segments and toss to combine.

5. For the dressing, whisk the ingredients together in a bowl and trickle over the salad.

6. Toss the salad well and serve, scattered with the reserved fennel fronds and dill.

· ·

THE LOWDOWN A sprinkling of toasted nuts adds a great crunch and texture to salads. Simply toast the nuts in a dry frying pan until fragrant and golden, tossing the pan to ensure they colour evenly.

· ·

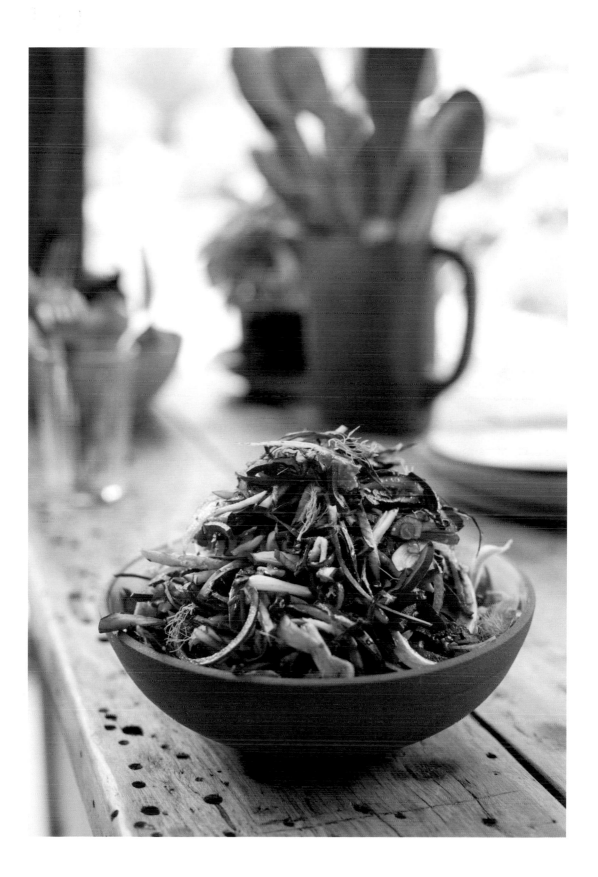

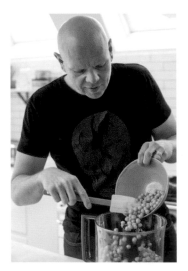

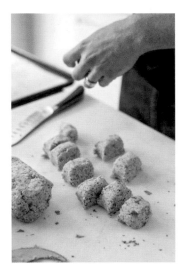

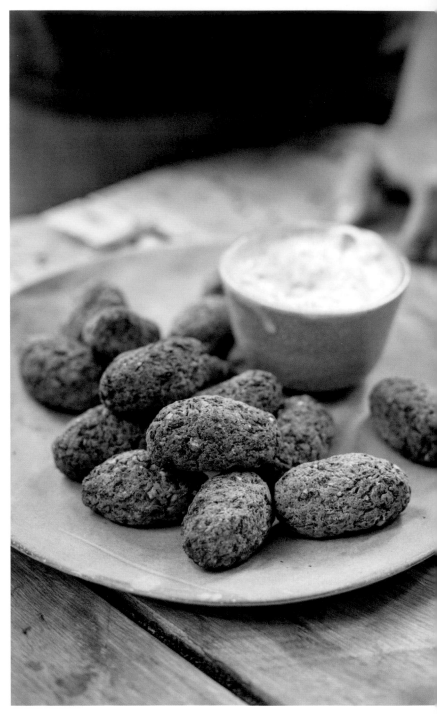

Baked falafel with tzatziki

Falafel seem like a healthy choice but usually they are deep-fried in oil. These, however, are baked for a lower calorie and lower fat version that still delivers a crisp outer layer and soft interior. For a more substantial meal, and to up your veg intake, serve them with a salad and the pickled beetroot hummus on page 180.

Makes: 18

Calories: 75 per falafel

---

1 tsp olive oil
2 medium-small onions
    (200g in total), finely diced
2 x 400g tins chickpeas,
    rinsed and drained
4 garlic cloves, grated
3 tsp ground cumin
2 tsp ground coriander
2 tsp flaky sea salt
30g coriander leaves, roughly
    chopped
30g flat-leaf parsley leaves,
    roughly chopped
40g plain flour
Freshly ground black pepper
Olive oil spray

For the tzatziki
200ml natural yoghurt (0% fat)
140g piece of cucumber, grated
1 small garlic clove, finely grated
2 tbsp mint leaves, finely chopped
A pinch of sea salt
A pinch of granulated sweetener

1. Preheat the oven to fan 230°C/gas 8 and line a baking tray with baking parchment.

2. Heat the olive oil in small non-stick frying pan over a medium heat. Add the onions and cook for about 10 minutes or until softened and starting to brown, adding a splash of water if they start to stick. Remove from the heat and leave to cool.

3. Put the onions, chickpeas, garlic, spices, salt, chopped herbs, flour and some pepper in a food processor. Pulse until the mixture is fairly smooth, stopping every so often to scrape down the sides with a spatula. You want to retain some texture but the paste should be able to hold together.

4. Divide the mixture into 18 equal pieces and shape into patties. Place on the prepared baking tray and spray the patties with 10 sprays of oil. Cook on the top shelf of the oven for 20–25 minutes or until golden brown.

5. Meanwhile, make the tzatziki. Put the yoghurt into a small bowl. Squeeze the grated cucumber to remove excess liquid, then add to the yoghurt with the garlic, mint, salt and sweetener. Mix well.

6. Lower the oven setting to fan 180°C/gas 4 and move the tray of falafel to the bottom shelf of the oven. Bake for a further 20–25 minutes or until cooked through. Sprinkle with a little salt and serve with the tzatziki.

Chickpea and spinach curry

Eating less meat is an easy way to cut back on calories, and chickpeas are a fantastic alternative as they're both sustaining and a good source of protein. They readily take on other flavours too, so they are great in a curry. Serve this on its own as a main dish, or as part of a selection of curries if you're feeding a crowd.

Serves: 4

Calories: 380 per serving

1 tbsp vegetable oil
2 medium onions, finely chopped
6 garlic cloves, finely grated
6cm piece of ginger, finely grated
2 long green chillies, finely
    chopped
1 tsp ground cumin
1 tsp ground coriander
2 tsp garam masala
1 tsp ground turmeric
1 tsp flaky sea salt
2 tbsp tomato purée
2 x 400g tins chopped tomatoes
400ml fresh vegetable stock
2 x 400g tins chickpeas, rinsed
    and drained
150g baby spinach

To finish
4 tbsp natural yoghurt (0% fat)
Sprigs of coriander

1. Heat the oil in a large non-stick saucepan over a high heat. Add the onions and cook for 5 minutes or until they are starting to brown, adding a splash of water if they start to stick.

2. Add the garlic, ginger and chillies and cook for about 2 minutes. Sprinkle in the spices and salt and cook, stirring, for 1 minute. Stir in the tomato purée and cook for another minute.

3. Add the tinned tomatoes, stock and chickpeas, bring to a simmer and cook for 20–30 minutes until the sauce thickens. If it gets too thick, loosen with a splash of boiling water.

4. When ready to serve, stir through the spinach and cook briefly, just until it wilts.

5. Divide the curry between warmed bowls and top each portion with a dollop of yoghurt and a sprig of coriander to serve.

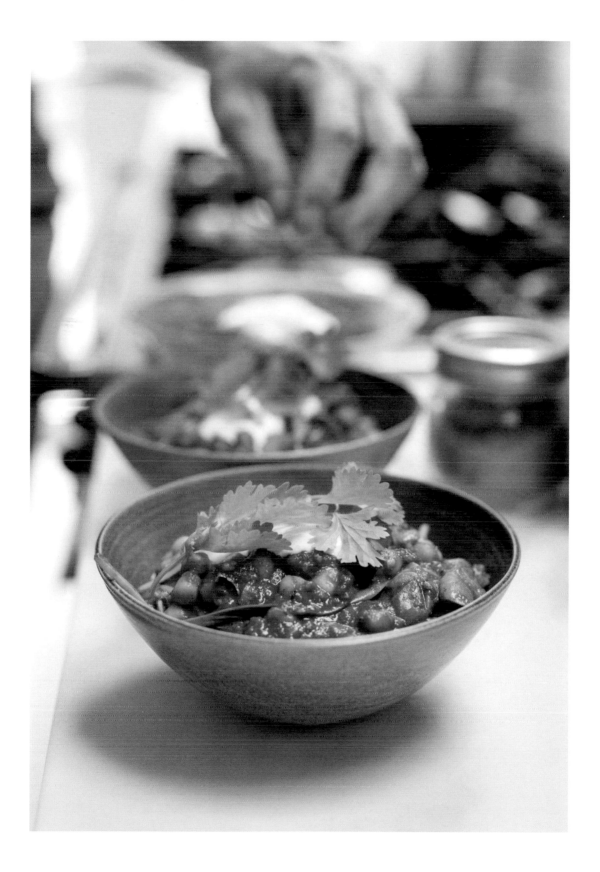

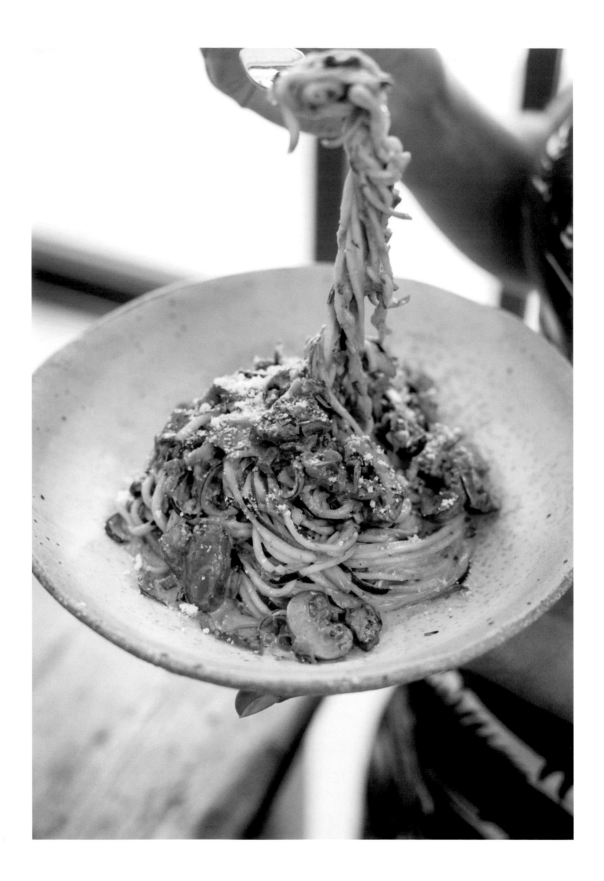

Creamy wild mushroom courgetti

Using courgette strands instead of pasta significantly reduces calories, while upping your veg intake. Once you give it a go, I promise you'll love it! Using dried porcini mushrooms in this sauce creates a wonderful deep, savoury hit.

Serves: 4

Calories: 320 per serving

1kg courgettes, spiralized
50g dried porcini mushrooms
250ml just-boiled water
1 tbsp olive oil
1 onion, finely diced
4 garlic cloves, finely chopped
250g chestnut mushrooms, thickly sliced
1 tbsp thyme leaves
300ml light single cream alternative
100g porcini and truffle paste (or umami paste)
2 tbsp flat-leaf parsley leaves, finely chopped
Flaky sea salt and freshly ground black pepper
20g grated Parmesan, to finish

1. Put the spiralized courgettes into a bowl and sprinkle generously with salt. Mix well with your hands, then leave to stand and wilt for 20 minutes. Drain in a colander, patting the courgette firmly with kitchen paper to remove all excess water and salt.

2. Meanwhile, put the dried porcini into a small bowl and pour on the just-boiled water. Cover with cling film and leave to soak for 15 minutes.

3. Heat the olive oil in a large non-stick sauté pan. Add the onion and cook over a medium heat for 4–5 minutes until softened, adding a splash of water if it starts to stick. Stir in the garlic and cook for 2 minutes.

4. Add the chestnut mushrooms, then strain the porcini soaking liquid into the pan. Chop the rehydrated porcini and add them to the pan with the thyme leaves, 'cream' and porcini and truffle paste. Lower the heat to a simmer and cook for 5 minutes or until the sauce thickens slightly.

5. Stir through the parsley, then add the courgetti and toss to coat. Season with salt and pepper and cook over a medium heat for 2 minutes. Transfer to warmed bowls and sprinkle with the Parmesan.

THE LOWDOWN Adding a little porcini and truffle paste gives the dish a really luxurious umami flavour with very few extra calories.

Stuffed peppers

When you're watching your weight, feeling satisfied by a meal helps to keep you motivated. In the filling for these stuffed peppers, the melting mozzarella tastes utterly decadent and cauliflower replaces the usual rice, reducing the calories without you even noticing.

Serves: 2 as a main, 4 as a starter

Calories: 320 per serving as a main
160 as a starter

2 large yellow or red peppers
½ tbsp light olive oil
1 red onion, finely diced
2 garlic cloves, finely grated
1 small yellow pepper, cored, deseeded and diced
100g courgette, diced
80g button mushrooms, sliced
1 tbsp tomato purée
½ tsp dried oregano
100g tomatoes, diced
40g pitted kalamata olives, sliced
120ml fresh vegetable stock
150g cauliflower 'rice' (see page 18)
2 handfuls of basil leaves, finely chopped
100g half-fat mozzarella, cut into 4 slices
Sea salt and freshly ground black pepper

1. Preheat the oven to fan 180°C/gas 4. Line a baking tray with baking parchment.

2. Halve the large peppers lengthways and remove the core and seeds. Place cut side up on the baking tray, shaving a thin sliver off the curved underside to ensure they lie steady, if necessary.

3. Heat the olive oil in a non-stick sauté pan then add the red onion and cook over a medium heat for 5–10 minutes, until softened and just starting to colour. Add the garlic and diced pepper and cook for 2 minutes. Add the courgette and mushrooms, stir through and cook for 2 minutes.

4. Stir in the tomato purée and cook for 1 minute. Add the dried oregano, tomatoes and olives and cook for 3–4 minutes, or until the tomatoes soften.

5. Pour in the veg stock, then add the cauliflower 'rice' and stir through. Cook for about 5 minutes, until the liquid has reduced a bit. Stir through the basil and season with salt and pepper.

6. Spoon the mixture into the pepper halves. Top each with a slice of mozzarella and bake on the middle shelf of the oven for 20–25 minutes or until the cheese is melted and golden brown. Serve hot.

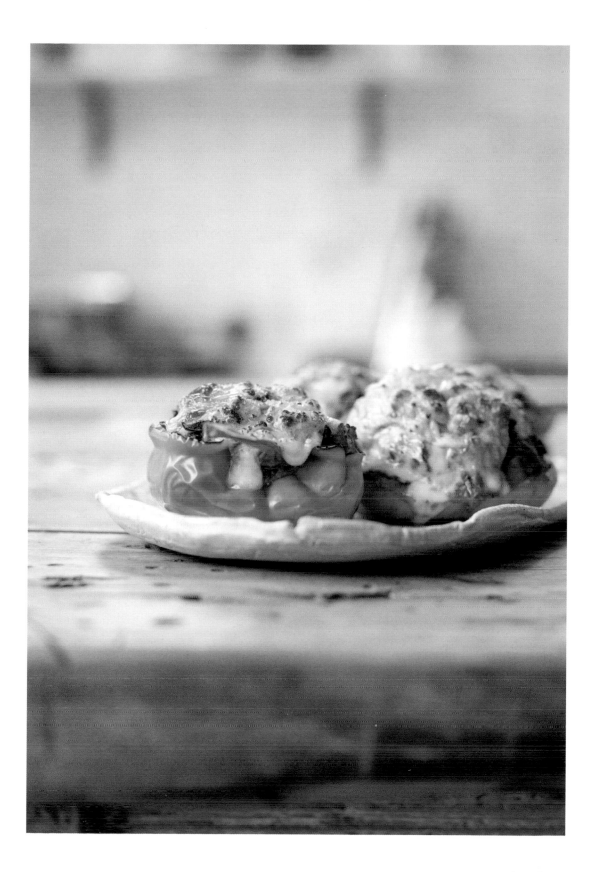

Courgette and ricotta pancakes

If you get yourself organised, these tasty pancakes can be ready in just 20 minutes. They are so simple and tasty. It just takes a bit of practice to cook them properly all the way through without over-browning the outside.

Serves: 2

Calories: 270 per serving

2 courgettes (250g in total), grated
50g self-raising flour
½ tsp baking powder
1 tsp ground cumin
1 large free-range egg, beaten
1 small garlic clove, finely grated
100g ricotta
2 tbsp finely chopped dill
A pinch of dried chilli flakes
Finely grated zest of 1 lemon
Sea salt and freshly ground black pepper
Olive oil spray

To serve
2 lemon wedges
40g mixed salad leaves (watercress, spinach etc.)
8 cherry tomatoes, halved

1. Squeeze the grated courgettes well to remove excess water, then tip into a bowl.

2. Add the flour, baking powder, cumin, egg, garlic, ricotta, chopped dill, chilli flakes and lemon zest. Season with salt and pepper and mix together well.

3. Heat a large non-stick frying pan over a medium heat and spray the pan 10 times with oil.

4. Drop 6 large spoonfuls of batter into the pan, spacing them well apart, and cook for 3–4 minutes on each side, until the pancakes are golden brown and cooked through. (If your pan isn't large enough to take 6 pancakes, cook them in batches.)

5. Serve 3 pancakes each, with a leafy salad on the side and lemon wedges for squeezing.

THE LOWDOWN Grated vegetables give these savoury pancakes a lovely light texture. They're great for packing up and taking to work for lunch, or as a quick snack if you're on the go.

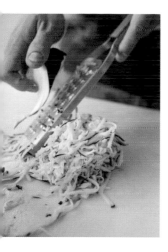

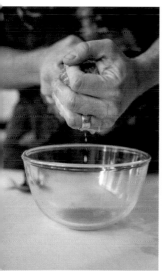

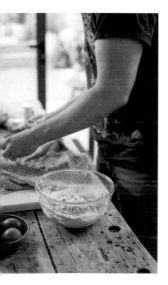

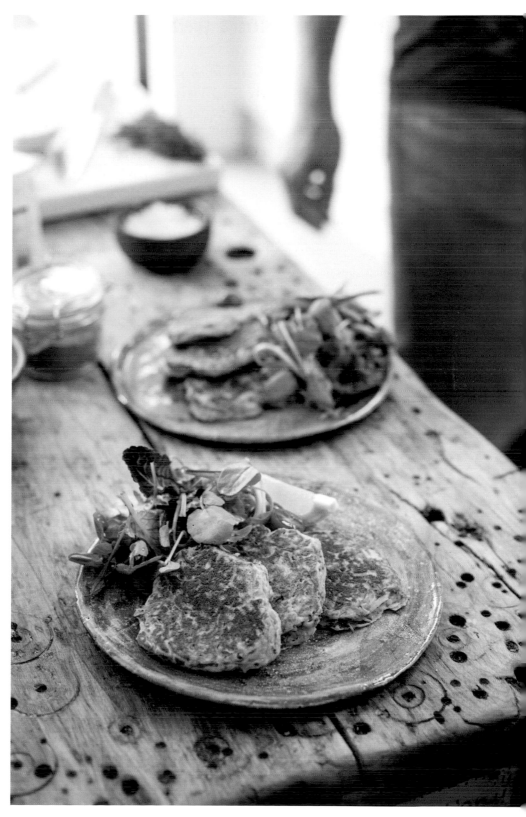

Toasted cabbage tart with ricotta and lemon

Cabbage is a robust ingredient – bold enough to take centre-stage in this beautiful tart. Reduced-fat puff pastry gives a great, crunchy texture and feels a little bit luxurious when you're on a diet. Baby capers add a lovely piquancy to the filling.

Serves: 6

Calories: 340 per serving

320g ready-rolled light puff pastry
1 Savoy cabbage, cut into
   8 wedges
1 tbsp semi-skimmed milk
200g ricotta
1 large free-range egg
3 garlic cloves, finely grated
20g grated Parmesan
Finely grated zest and juice of
   1 lemon
2 tbsp baby capers
Olive oil spray
Sea salt and freshly ground
   black pepper

1. Unroll the pastry onto a baking tray lined with baking parchment and score a border 2cm in from the edge all the way round. Prick the pastry within the border with a fork. Chill in the fridge for 1 hour.

2. Blanch the cabbage in boiling salted water for 3–4 minutes, until just tender. Drain in a colander and run under the cold tap to cool. Pat dry with kitchen paper. Preheat the oven to fan 220°C/gas 7.

3. Brush the pastry all over with the milk then cook on the top shelf of the oven for 15 minutes, rotating the tray halfway through cooking to ensure it colours evenly. Remove from the oven and turn the oven setting down to fan 140°C/gas 1.

4. Press the pastry within the border down and return to the oven for 25 minutes to crisp the base.

5. Meanwhile, in a bowl, beat together the ricotta, egg, garlic, Parmesan, lemon zest and juice, and season with salt and pepper.

6. Place the cabbage wedges on a metal tray and blowtorch them until lightly blackened and charred.

7. Remove the tart case from the oven. Increase the oven setting to fan 180°C/gas 4.

8. Spread the ricotta mixture in the tart case and lay the cabbage wedges on top. Sprinkle with capers, season with salt and pepper and spray 10–15 times with oil. Cook on the middle shelf of the oven for 15 minutes or until the cabbage is warmed through.

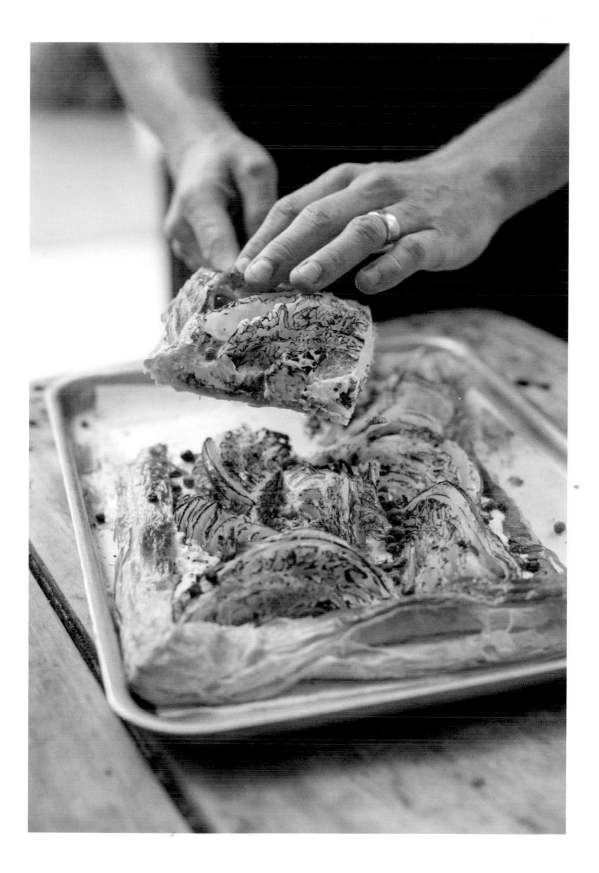

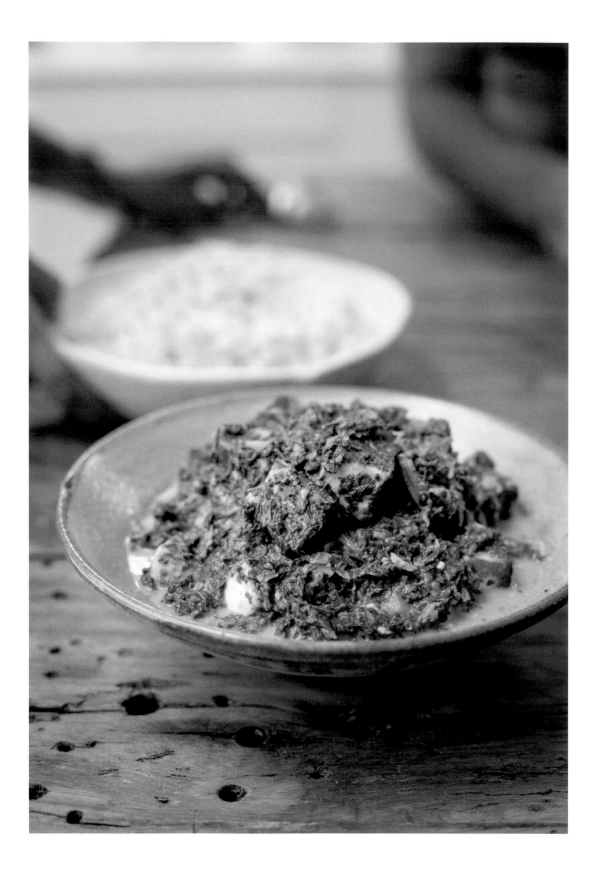

Spinach and paneer curry

Paneer is a lower fat cheese that holds its shape well during cooking, making it feel really substantial. There are some big flavours at work in this curry, which is great on its own, or with some saffron rice, or even a little poached chicken on the side.

Serves: 4

Calories: 550 per serving
335 without rice

250g paneer, cubed
¼ tsp ground turmeric
½ tsp flaky sea salt
Sunflower oil spray
½ tbsp vegetable oil
1 onion, finely diced
1 tsp cumin seeds
750g frozen spinach, defrosted
   and drained
200ml fresh vegetable stock
4 garlic cloves, finely chopped
2.5cm piece of ginger, finely grated
1 long green chilli, finely chopped
½ tsp garam masala
50ml light single cream
   alternative
200g tomatoes, diced
Sea salt and freshly ground
   black pepper

To serve (optional)
240g basmati rice, cooked
   with salt and a pinch of
   saffron strands

1. Place the paneer in a bowl and sprinkle over the turmeric and salt. Toss well, to coat the cheese all over.

2. Heat a large non-stick sauté pan over a high heat, then spray with oil 15 times. Add the paneer and cook for 5 minutes, tossing the pan frequently so the cheese cubes turn golden brown on all sides. Remove to a plate; set aside.

3. Add the vegetable oil to the pan. When hot, add the onion and cumin seeds and cook for 5 minutes or until the onion is starting to turn golden brown.

4. Meanwhile, roughly chop a third of the spinach. Put the remaining spinach into a food processor with the stock and blend until smooth.

5. Toss the garlic, ginger and chilli into the pan and cook, stirring, for 2 minutes, then add the garam masala and stir over the heat for another minute.

6. Add both the chopped and blended spinach. Return the paneer to the pan and stir through the 'cream' and tomatoes. Bring to a simmer and cook for 4–5 minutes until slightly thickened.

7. Season the curry to taste with salt and pepper and serve in warmed bowls, with saffron rice on the side, if you like.

Sweet potato and black bean burritos

I love making vegetables the heroes of a meal rather than banishing them to side-dish status. These burritos are packed with tasty veg, and there is so much going on in terms of texture and tastes, there's no way you'll miss the meat.

Serves: 4

Calories: 685 per serving

700g sweet potatoes (3 medium)
2 x 400g tins black beans,
    rinsed and drained
50g walnuts, toasted
2 tsp hot smoked paprika
1 tsp dried Italian herb mix
1 tsp garlic powder
1 tsp onion powder
Sea salt and freshly ground
    black pepper

For the chipotle yoghurt
2 tsp chipotle paste
100g Greek yoghurt (0% fat)

To assemble
4 large corn (or wheat) tortillas
100g iceberg lettuce, shredded
200g carrots, grated
200g raw beetroot, peeled
    and grated
1 ripe, small avocado, peeled
    and quartered

1. Preheat the oven to fan 180°C/gas 4.

2. Prick the sweet potatoes all over with a fork and put on a small baking tray. Bake for 50–60 minutes or until soft all the way through. Remove from the oven and allow to cool. Turn off the oven. Scoop out the flesh from the sweet potatoes into a large bowl.

3. Put half the black beans into a food processor with the walnuts and blend until smooth. Add to the sweet potato flesh, with the remaining black beans, paprika, dried herb mix, garlic powder and onion powder. Season with salt and pepper and mix well.

4. Line a baking tray with baking parchment. Divide the mixture into 4 portions and shape into logs, about 15 x 7 x 2cm, on the lined tray. Flatten them slightly and chill in the fridge to firm up for 2 hours.

5. Heat the oven again to fan 180°C/gas 4. Cook the sweet potato patties on the middle shelf of the oven for 50 minutes.

6. Meanwhile, mix the chipotle paste and yoghurt together in a bowl. When the patties are cooked, place the tortillas in the oven for 1 minute until warm but still pliable.

7. Spread each tortilla with a big spoonful of the chipotle yoghurt and place a sweet potato patty in the middle. Top with lettuce, carrot and beetroot. Slice an avocado quarter in half and lay both pieces on top, then roll the tortilla around the filling tightly. Slice in half to serve.

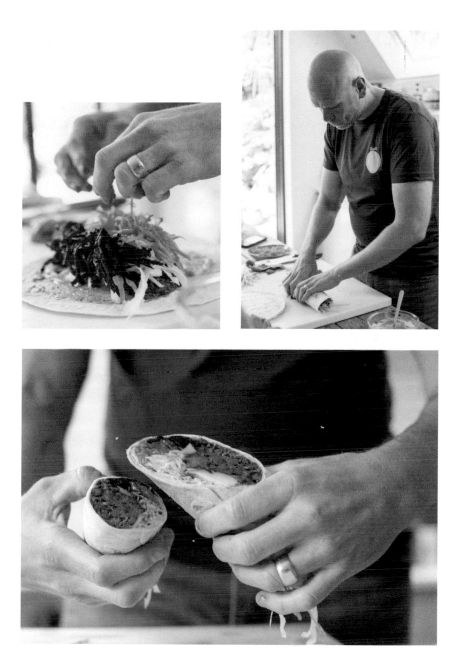

THE LOWDOWN Sweet potatoes have much more flavour than regular potatoes and more fibre too. Not only that, they taste amazing, count towards your 'five-a-day' and their flesh is a fantastic orange colour.

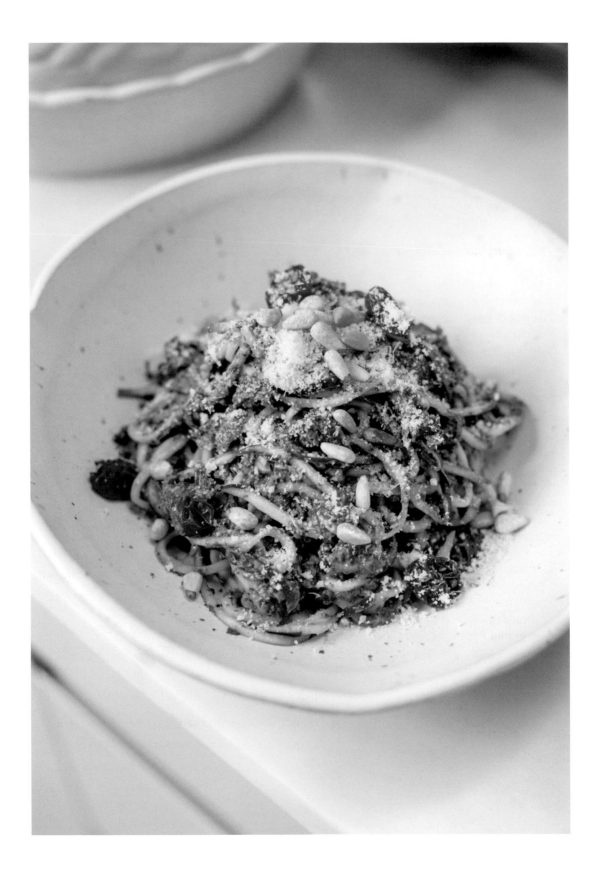

Spinach and basil pesto courgetti

A simple, fresh and filling take on the classic Italian pasta and pesto combination. Don't be afraid of the spiralizer – it's a versatile, easy-to-use bit of kit. You'll love it, I promise, and soon you'll be spiralizing all sorts of veg.

Serves: 2

Calories: 245 per serving

180g cherry tomatoes, halved
Olive oil spray
1 tsp dried oregano
500g courgettes, spiralized
2 tbsp light single cream
    alternative
Flaky sea salt and freshly ground
    black pepper

For the spinach and basil pesto
150g baby spinach
30g basil leaves
1 garlic clove, finely grated
1 tbsp extra virgin olive oil
Finely grated zest of 1 lemon
2 tbsp fresh vegetable stock
    or water
½ tsp freshly grated nutmeg

To finish
10g pine nuts
A small handful of basil leaves,
    shredded
2 tsp grated Parmesan

1. Preheat the oven to fan 140°C/gas 1. Line an oven tray with baking parchment.

2. Place the cherry tomatoes, cut side up, on the prepared tray and spray 10 times with oil. Sprinkle each tomato with a little oregano, salt and pepper. Cook on the middle shelf of the oven for 1¼ hours, then set aside to cool.

3. Meanwhile, for the pesto, put all the ingredients into a jug blender or food processor, add some salt and pepper and blitz until smooth.

4. Toast the pine nuts for the garnish in a small, dry pan for 30 seconds, then tip onto a plate and set aside.

5. Put the spiralized courgettes into a bowl and sprinkle generously with salt. Mix well with your hands, then leave to stand and wilt for 20 minutes. Drain in a colander, patting the courgette firmly with kitchen paper to remove all excess water and salt.

6. Tip the spiralized courgettes into a large pan and add the pesto and 'cream'. Stir well to coat with the sauce and cook over a medium heat for 2 minutes, then fold through the roasted tomatoes.

7. Divide the courgetti between warmed serving bowls and sprinkle with the shredded basil, Parmesan and toasted pine nuts.

Mediterranean puff pastry tart

Pastry seems like a real treat when you're cutting down on calories, but you don't need much to feel like you've eaten something special. The key to this tart is to pack the topping with flavour – so the veggies are heavy on the garlic and herbs, and the addition of goat's cheese brings a satisfying, rich creaminess.

Serves: 4

Calories: 400 per serving

280g ready-rolled light puff pastry
200g baby courgettes, cut into
    1.5cm slices
1 large red pepper, cored,
    deseeded and cut into
    2cm chunks
1 large yellow pepper, cored,
    deseeded and cut into
    2cm chunks
1 red onion, cut into 2cm chunks
4 garlic cloves, sliced
2 sprigs of rosemary, leaves
    picked and finely chopped
4 sprigs of thyme, leaves picked
Olive oil spray
1 tbsp semi-skimmed milk
100g cherry tomatoes, halved
75g goat's cheese, crumbled
Sea salt and freshly ground
    black pepper

1. Using a sharp knife, trim the sheet of puff pastry to 25 x 28cm. Place it on a baking tray lined with baking parchment and score a border 2cm in from the edge all the way round. Prick the pastry within the margin, using a fork. Leave to rest in the fridge for about 1 hour. Meanwhile, preheat the oven to fan 220°C/gas 7.

2. Put the courgettes, peppers and red onion into a large bowl. Add the garlic and herbs and season generously with salt and pepper. Line a large baking tray with baking parchment, lay the veg out on it and spray 15–20 times with oil.

3. Brush the puff pastry all over with the milk and sprinkle with a little salt. Cook on the middle shelf of the oven, with the veg tray on the top shelf above, for 15 minutes, rotating both trays halfway through to ensure even colouring. Remove both trays from the oven and turn the setting down to fan 140°C/gas 1. Set the veg aside.

4. Press the inside of the pastry down and return to the oven for 25 minutes to get a super crispy base.

5. Take the tart case out of the oven and turn the setting up to fan 180°C/gas 4. Tip the roasted veg into the tart case, scatter over the cherry tomatoes and goat's cheese and season with salt and pepper. Bake for 20–25 minutes until the veg are cooked through and the cheese is softening and colouring at the edges. Cut the tart into quarters to serve.

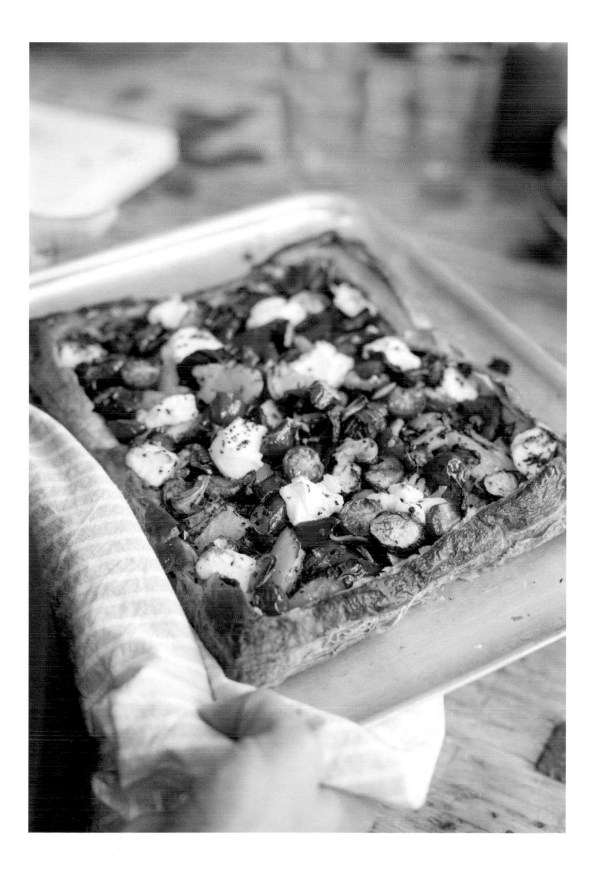

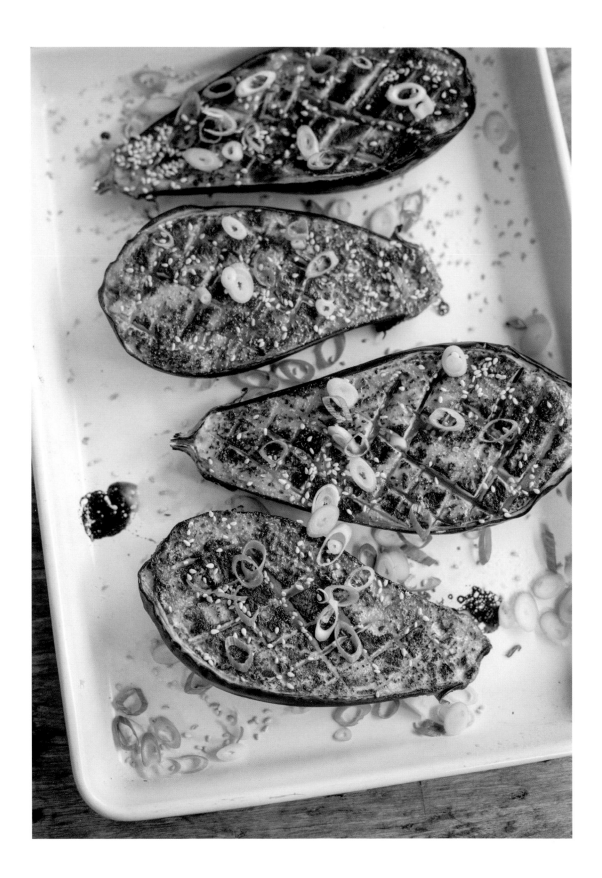

Japanese miso aubergine

Keep your palate entertained when you're on a diet and you won't even realise you are cutting back on calories. This sweet and sticky miso glaze works perfectly with the meaty aubergine, and the scattering of sesame seeds adds a subtle crunch.

Serves: 2 as a main, 4 as a side

Calories: 220 per serving as a main 110 as a side

2 aubergines (300g each)
Sunflower oil spray
½ tsp flaky sea salt
1 spring onion, finely sliced on an angle
½ tsp sesame seeds, toasted

For the miso glaze
2 tbsp white miso paste
2 tbsp mirin
2 tbsp caster sugar
2.5cm piece of ginger, finely grated

1. Preheat the oven to fan 180°C/gas 4.

2. Halve the aubergines lengthways then, using a small sharp knife, deeply score the flesh of each half in a criss-cross pattern. Place on an oven tray. Spray each aubergine half 5 or 6 times with oil, then sprinkle with a little flaky salt. Bake on the top shelf of the oven for 25 minutes.

3. Meanwhile, for the miso glaze, mix the miso, mirin, sugar and grated ginger together in a small bowl.

4. Remove the tray of aubergines from the oven and leave to cool for 2 minutes. Pour off any excess liquid released by the aubergines.

5. Preheat the grill to medium-high.

6. Spoon the miso glaze generously on top of each aubergine half and spread evenly to the edges. Grill the aubergines for 5–7 minutes or until golden brown and caramelised.

7. Sprinkle the spring onion and toasted sesame seeds over the aubergine halves and serve.

Egg-fried wild rice

This lighter version of everyone's favourite egg-fried rice is packed with texture and flavour – and is virtually fat-free. Wild rice has a great, nutty taste and is slightly chewy, which brings another layer of interest to an already exciting dish. You can use whatever veg you like – you could even stir-fry some chopped prawns or strips of chicken breast if you're not serving it up to vegetarians.

Serves: 4

Calories: 570 per serving

30g dried shiitake mushrooms
250ml just-boiled water
1 tsp toasted sesame oil
2 garlic cloves, finely chopped
1 green pepper, cored, deseeded
    and diced
75g oyster mushrooms, roughly
    torn into pieces
75g small chestnut mushrooms,
    sliced
2 x 250g packets ready-cooked
    long-grain and wild rice
100g tinned sweetcorn, drained
100g frozen peas
4 spring onions, finely sliced
2 tbsp light soy sauce
80g bean sprouts
Freshly ground white pepper

For the rolled egg
2 large free-range eggs
1 tsp vegetable oil
Flaky sea salt and freshly ground
    white pepper

To finish
½ tsp black sesame seeds

1. Put the dried shiitake into a bowl and pour on the 250ml just-boiled water. Cover with cling film and leave to soak for 20 minutes. Drain the shiitake, reserving the liquor, and chop roughly; set aside.

2. Meanwhile, prepare the rolled egg: beat the eggs in a bowl with a good pinch each of salt and white pepper. Heat the oil in a non-stick wok over a high heat, swirling it around the bottom and sides of the wok to coat.

3. When the oil is hot, pour in the eggs and swirl the wok around until a thin layer of egg begins to form. Lifting the wok off the heat, keep swirling it until there is no runny egg left. Put the wok back on the heat for 30 seconds or so to cook the egg, and then take it off again. Run a rubber spatula around the edges to release the cooked egg, then tip the wok upside down over a board so the omelette falls out onto the board. Roll up the omelette while still warm and set aside.

4. Return the wok to a high heat, add the sesame oil and garlic, and stir-fry for 30 seconds. Add the green pepper and stir-fry for 2 minutes.

5. Next add the oyster, chestnut and rehydrated shiitake mushrooms and stir-fry for 2–3 minutes.

6. Crumble in the ready-cooked rice, strain in the reserved mushroom soaking liquor and stir-fry for 2–3 minutes.

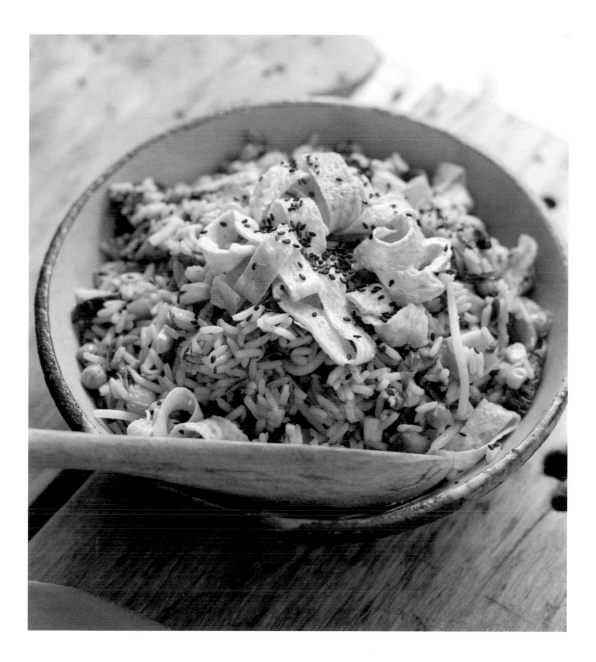

7. Add the sweetcorn, peas, spring onions and soy sauce. Stir-fry for 2 minutes, then toss in the bean sprouts and add a generous pinch of white pepper. Stir-fry for another minute.

8. Divide the stir-fry between warmed bowls. Slice the rolled omelette and arrange on top. Finish with a sprinkling of sesame seeds.

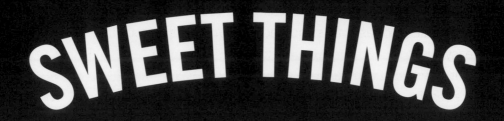

SWEET THINGS

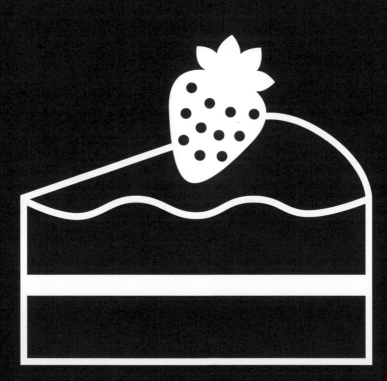

Losing weight is so much about changing your mindset – taking the first step and then sticking with it. But for many, cutting out daily treats such as that afternoon slice of cake with your cup of tea is a difficult step. Chocolate, cookies, cakes and puddings are comfort foods and I know just how easy it is to munch through a packet of biscuits without even thinking about it! But, although it can be tough at times, you have to commit to losing weight to get the results. To help when sugar cravings strike, I've come up with lower calorie versions of some of my favourite sweet things and I'd like to share them with you.

The recipes in this chapter make use of a lot of fruit (and some veg!), which introduces a lovely natural sweetness, without the empty calories of refined sugar. I have also used some low-fat alternatives, swapping full-fat milk for skimmed and double cream for light cream alternatives, and I make use of sweeteners to reduce the amount of regular sugar, or replace it altogether. Simple changes like this can instantly cut down on calories without compromising on taste.

There are some intense flavours at play here, such as a splash of aromatic rosewater in my creamy rice pudding on page 219, ground mace in the French apple tarts (page 220), a little cardamom in the courgette cake on page 232 and beautifully contrasting coffee and chocolate in the custard pots on page 227.

Complementary textures help make a really satisfying treat too. Try the Vanilla and strawberry cheesecake (page 231) with its creamy quark topping and crisp biscuit base, or the generously spiced Carrot cake (page 235) with its smooth, rich frosting.

It is possible to enjoy the occasional delicious pudding while watching your weight – it's all about moderation and balance, and looking for clever ways to pack in flavour without piling on the calories. You really can have your cake and eat it, only perhaps less often than you used to!

Baked Bramley apples and custard

Bramleys are the perfect apples for baking as they retain their flavour well and have a lovely, fluffy texture. This is such an easy pud, not least because you don't have to make the custard from scratch. The deep spices and amaretti biscuits give it some really big flavours.

Serves: 4

Calories: 240 per serving

75g sachet low-fat instant
    custard powder
400ml skimmed milk
4 large Bramley apples
40g amaretti biscuits, crushed
Finely grated zest of 1 orange
30g raisins
1 tsp ground allspice
½ tsp ground ginger
½ tsp ground cardamom
1 tbsp soft light brown sugar

1. Preheat the oven to fan 160°C/gas 3.

2. Tip the custard powder into a large heatproof jug. Heat the milk in a small pan to just below the boil, then pour onto the custard powder, whisking until smooth. Set aside.

3. Prise out the core from each apple using an apple corer, making the hole a little bigger so that you have enough room for the filling.

4. In a small bowl, mix together the crushed amaretti biscuits, orange zest, raisins and spices.

5. Pour the custard into a small roasting dish. Place the apples in the dish and spoon the filling into the cavities. Bake in the oven for 20 minutes, then sprinkle with brown sugar and bake for a further 15 minutes.

6. Serve each stuffed baked apple with a portion of the hot custard.

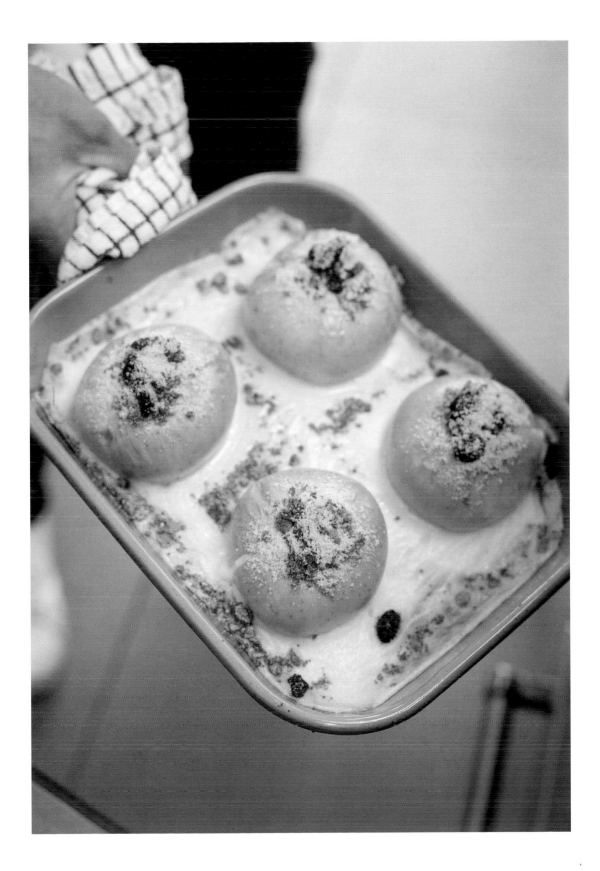

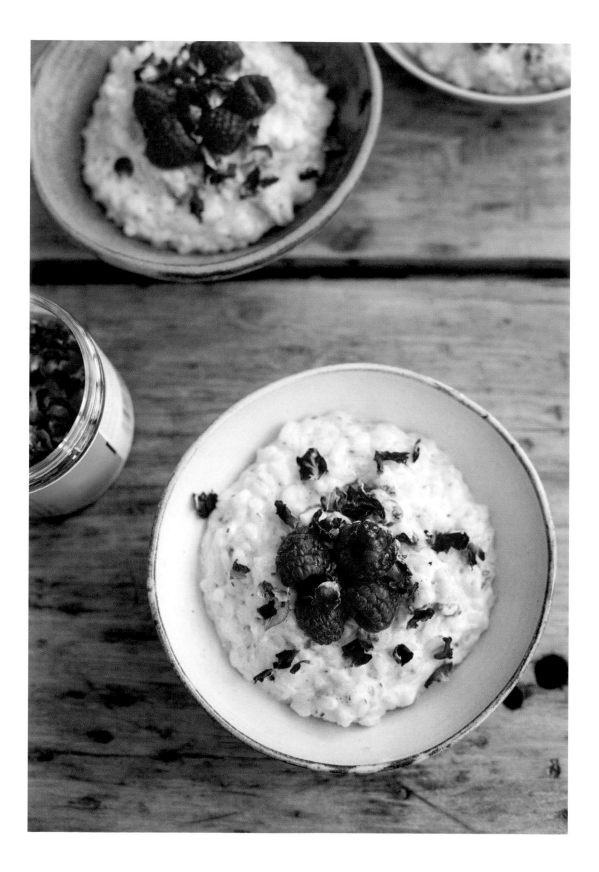

Rice pudding with rosewater and raspberries

This is a sophisticated low-cal version of the ever-popular creamy dessert. The exotic combination of rosewater, cardamom and vanilla ensures you won't need much of this indulgent pud to make you feel you've had something truly special.

Serves: 4

Calories: 290 per serving

200g pudding rice
800ml skimmed milk
4 tsp granulated sweetener
1 vanilla pod, split and
    seeds scraped
¼ tsp ground cardamom
200g raspberries
4–6 drops of rosewater, or to taste
60ml light single cream alternative
Dried rose petals, to finish
    (optional)

1. Preheat the oven to fan 190°C/gas 5.

2. Spread the rice out on a baking tray and toast in the oven for 15–20 minutes, until lightly browned.

3. Tip the rice into a medium saucepan and add the milk, sweetener, vanilla seeds and cardamom. Bring to a simmer over a medium heat.

4. Simmer gently, stirring frequently, for around 20–30 minutes until the rice is cooked and the mixture has thickened. To test, taste a few grains – they should be tender but still with a little bite. It's important to keep stirring regularly so the mixture doesn't stick to the bottom of the pan.

5. Set aside 16 raspberries to finish. Stir the remaining raspberries and the rosewater through the rice pudding, then stir through the 'cream'.

6. Serve the rice pudding in small serving bowls. Top each with 4 raspberries and a sprinkling of dried rose petals, if you like.

THE LOWDOWN Toasting the rice in the oven first gives an extra nutty layer of flavour. When you're on a diet, it's all about looking for ways to keep flavours interesting so you don't feel deprived.

French apple tarts with mace

Light, fruit-based puddings like this satisfy those sweet cravings while contributing to your 'five-a-day'. These tarts also work well with pears or plums.

Serves: 4

Calories: 325 per serving
265 without the yoghurt

200g ready-rolled light puff pastry
2 tbsp apricot jam
2 large sharp-tasting, green eating apples (300g in total)
1 tbsp semi-skimmed milk
2 tsp granulated sweetener
½ tsp ground cinnamon
½ tsp ground mace

For the yoghurt
125g Greek yoghurt (0% fat)
2 tbsp maple syrup
2 tsp chia seeds

1. For the yoghurt, in a small bowl, mix together the yoghurt, maple syrup and chia seeds. Cover and chill in the fridge for 2 hours, or overnight if you have the time.

2. Preheat the oven to fan 200°C/gas 6. Line a baking tray with baking parchment.

3. Cut the puff pastry into 4 equal pieces, about 10 x 13cm. Lay them on the lined baking tray.

4. Divide the jam between the 4 pieces of pastry and spread out with the back of a spoon, leaving a 1cm clear margin all the way around.

5. Quarter the apples, cut out the core, then slice thinly. Lay the apple slices, overlapping, on top of the jam. Brush the exposed edges of the pastry with the milk.

6. Mix together the sweetener, cinnamon and mace, then sprinkle liberally over each apple tart. Bake in the oven for 15–20 minutes until the pastry is golden brown and crispy.

7. Serve the apple tarts with a generous spoonful of the flavoured yoghurt on the side.

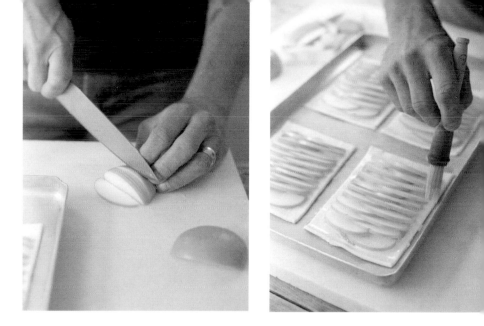

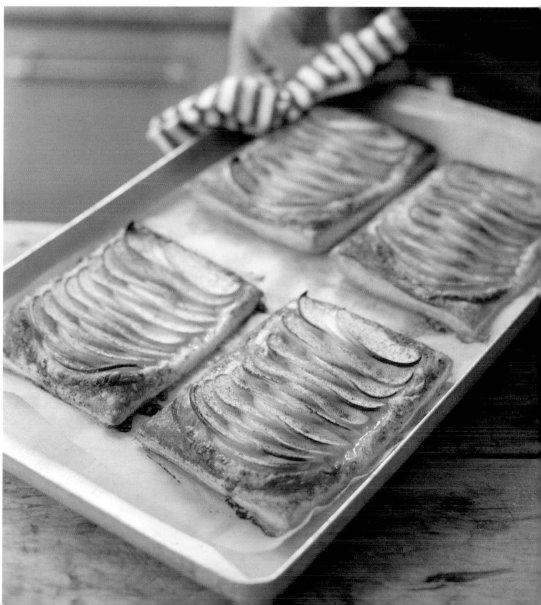

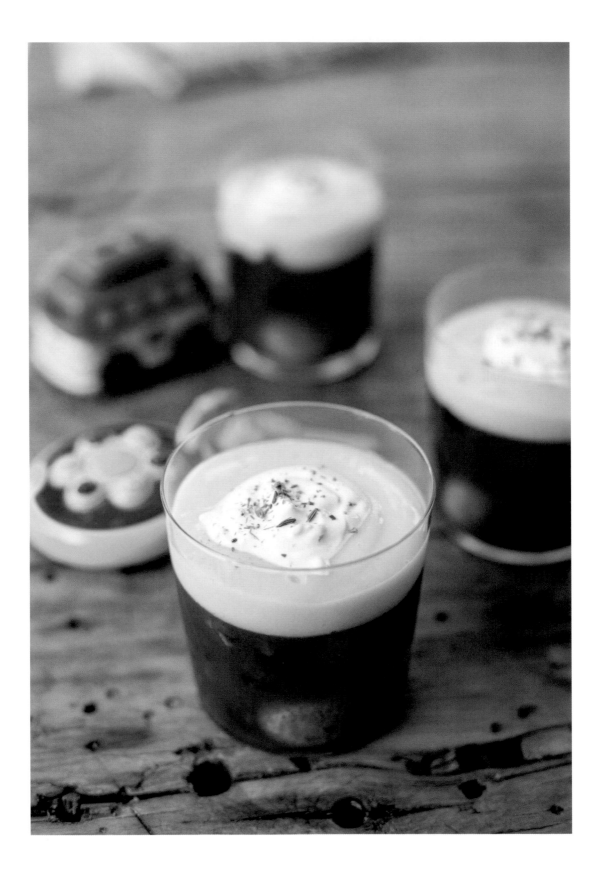

Jelly trifle with toasted fennel

Most jellies contain a lot of added sugar but this version uses cranberry juice and orange, for their natural sweetness as well as the all-important layers of flavour they add. Do check the calorie content of the sponge fingers as they can vary quite a lot – look for those that are 25 calories each.

Serves: 4

Calories: 140 per serving

6 sheets of leaf gelatine
600ml no-added-sugar cranberry
   juice
8 basil leaves, chopped
   (save the stalks)
Finely grated zest and juice
   of 1 small orange
6 sponge fingers, halved
300g mixed berries
200ml low-fat custard

For the topping
75ml half-fat crème fraîche
½ tsp granulated sweetener
1 tsp fennel seeds, toasted
   and crushed

1. Place the gelatine in a shallow dish, cover with cold water and leave to soak for about 5 minutes.

2. Meanwhile, heat the cranberry juice with the reserved basil stalks in a saucepan over a medium heat. When it begins to simmer, take off the heat. Immediately lift the gelatine out of the water and add it to the hot liquid, stirring until dissolved, then add the orange zest, orange juice and basil leaves.

3. Leave to cool, then pass the mixture through a sieve into a jug.

4. Place 3 sponge-finger halves in each of four 400ml serving glasses. Pour on just enough liquid jelly to cover them and leave to set in the fridge for 1½ hours. (Keep the rest of the jelly at room temperature, so it stays liquid.)

5. Once the jelly has set, spoon the berries evenly on top. Carefully pour on the rest of the liquid jelly and place in the fridge to set for at least 5 hours, ideally overnight.

6. For the topping, whisk the crème fraîche with the sweetener and half the toasted fennel seeds.

7. When the jellies have set, spoon the custard on top of them to cover completely. Add a spoonful of crème fraîche and sprinkle with the remaining toasted fennel seeds to serve.

Frozen red fruit yoghurt and basil

This is like an instant, frozen, fruity ice cream – full of flavour and texture but fat-free, as it uses 0% Greek yoghurt and frozen bananas instead of cream. Basil pairs really well with berries, but you could also use fresh mint.

Serves: 2

Calories: 175 per serving

250g Greek yoghurt (0% fat)
250g frozen mixed berries
50g frozen sliced banana
1 tbsp agave
12 basil leaves

To finish
50g mixed fresh berries
Freshly ground black pepper
(optional)

1. Using a jug blender or food processor, blend the yoghurt, frozen berries, frozen banana, agave and basil leaves together until smooth. The mixture will be very thick so you may need to scrape down the sides with a rubber spatula.

2. Spoon the frozen yoghurt mix into small serving bowls and serve straight away, topped with the fresh berries. A little pepper on top won't go amiss.

THE LOWDOWN Frozen berries are great to have on hand for instant puddings and smoothies. Frozen mango would also work well – just remember that it is higher in natural fruit sugar.

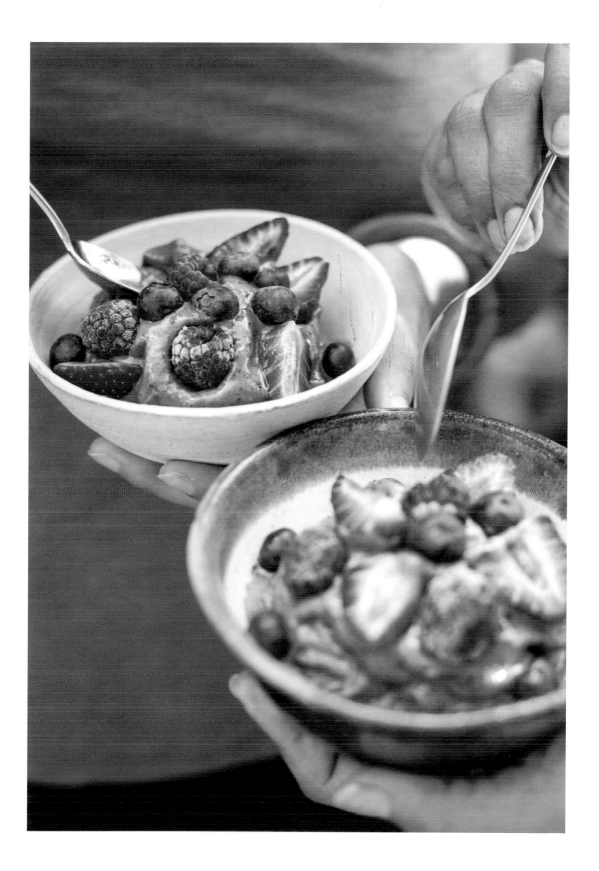

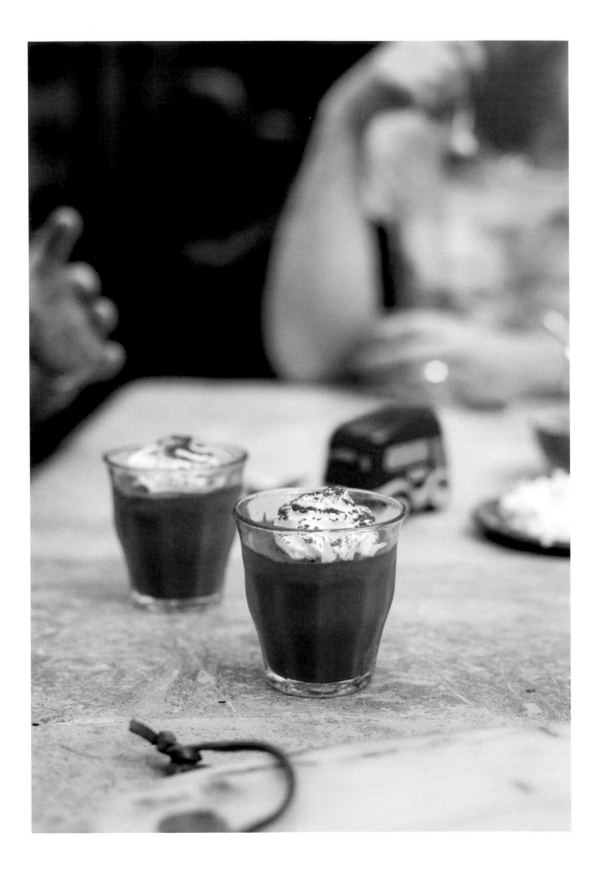

Coffee and chocolate custard pots

This easy, no-fuss mocha dessert is ideal to make in advance and it tastes like a truly indulgent treat. The chocolate, espresso, cardamom and orange zest introduce some luxurious layers of intense flavour. Using ready-made low-fat custard as the base instead of double cream is a clever time-saver, as well as a calorie-saver!

Serves: 4

Calories: 155 per serving

400ml low-fat custard
60g dark chocolate (70% cocoa
    solids), broken into pieces
40ml strong espresso coffee
Finely grated zest of ½ orange
¼ tsp ground cardamom

To finish
25ml squirty light cream
¼ tsp cocoa powder

1. Gently heat the custard in a saucepan over a medium heat. Add the chocolate followed by the espresso, orange zest and cardamom. Stir until the chocolate has melted, then pass the mixture through a sieve into a jug.

2. Pour into four 125ml individual pots or serving bowls and place in the fridge to firm up for at least 3 hours – it won't set completely firm.

3. Remove from the fridge and top with some light squirty cream and a dusting of cocoa.

Tropical cheesecake pots

You can make this easy dessert at any time, since tropical fruits are available all year round. Quark is a low-fat dairy product that has a wonderful acidity; here it balances the sweetness of the fruit, while adding a creamy texture to the topping.

Serves: 4

Calories: 255 per serving

2 sheets of leaf gelatine
4 light digestive biscuits
Finely grated zest and juice
    of 1 lime
2 tbsp granulated sweetener
150g light cream cheese
250g quark
150g Greek yoghurt with honey
1 vanilla pod, split and seeds
    scraped

For the topping
150g mango, diced
100g pineapple, diced
1 large passion fruit, halved

1. Place the gelatine leaves in a shallow dish, cover with cold water and leave to soak for about 5 minutes.

2. Meanwhile, put the biscuits into a strong plastic bag and bash with a rolling pin to crush to crumbs. Divide between four small glasses.

3. Heat the lime juice and 1 tbsp sweetener in a small pan over a medium heat. When hot, take the pan off the heat. Immediately lift the gelatine out of its water and add it to the hot liquid, stirring until dissolved. Leave to cool until barely tepid.

4. In a large bowl, whisk the cream cheese, quark, yoghurt, lime zest, remaining 1 tbsp sweetener and the vanilla seeds together until smooth. Whisk in the cooled gelatine mixture.

5. Spoon on top of the biscuit bases in the serving glasses and spread evenly. Chill in the fridge to set for at least 2 hours.

6. For the topping, mix the mango and pineapple together and spoon on top of the cheesecake pots. Finish with the passion fruit pulp and seeds.

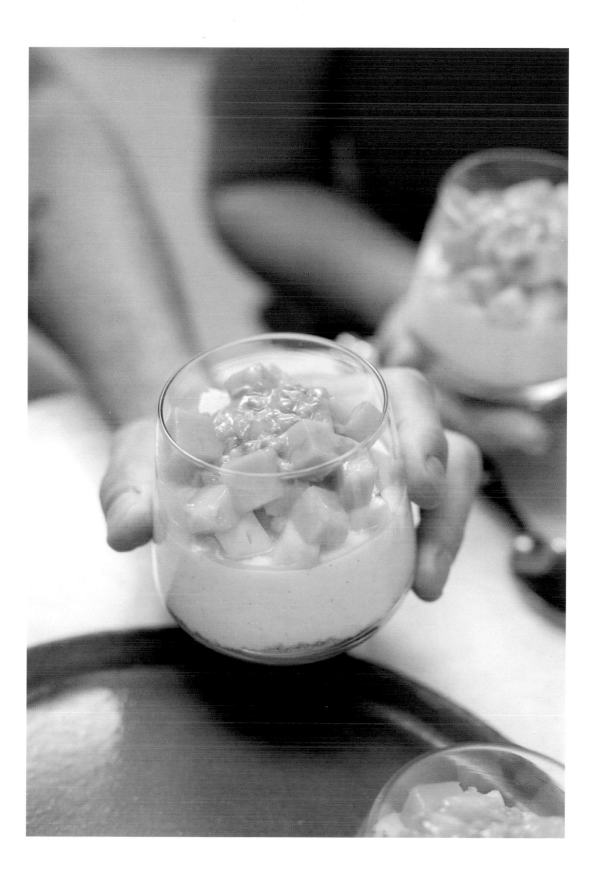

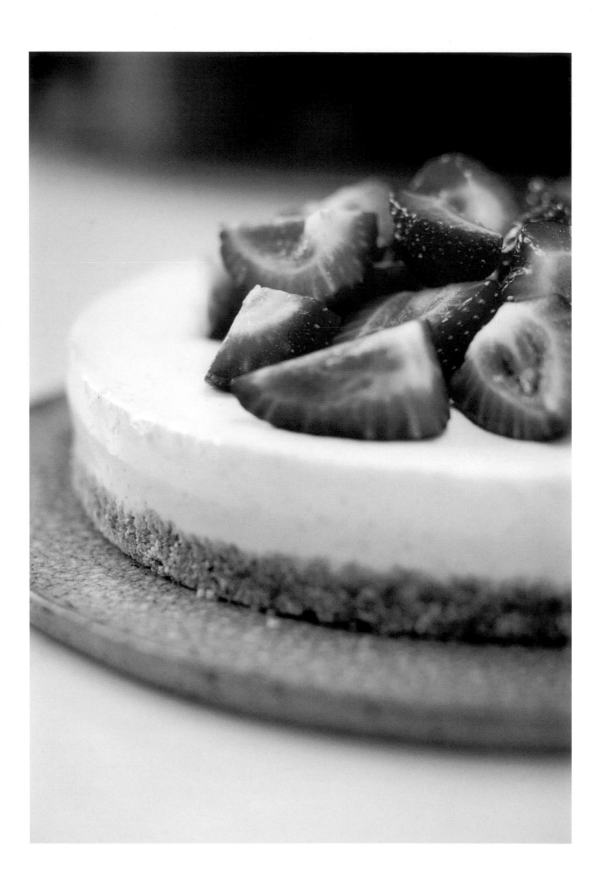

Vanilla and strawberry cheesecake

For the base, this cheesecake uses amaretti and light rich tea biscuits instead of the usual digestive biscuits – so it's lower in cals but also has much more flavour. The topping is deliciously light and creamy as it's made from quark – a great ingredient for lower calorie desserts. You can keep the cheesecake in the fridge for up to 4 days.

Serves: 10–12

Calories: 165–140 per serving

For the biscuit base
75g amaretti biscuits, crushed
75g light rich tea biscuits, crushed
A pinch of sea salt
50g half-fat margarine, melted

For the filling
3 sheets of leaf gelatine
Finely grated zest of 1 lemon and
    the juice of 2 lemons (70ml)
4 tbsp granulated sweetener
500g quark
250g ricotta
2 vanilla pods, split and seeds
    scraped

For the topping
200g strawberries, halved

....

THE LOWDOWN Quark is naturally low in fat and sugar, yet high in protein – helping you to feel full for longer.

....

1. Place the gelatine leaves for the filling in a shallow dish, cover with cold water and leave to soak for about 5 minutes.

2. For the base, in a bowl, stir together the crushed amaretti and rich tea biscuits with a pinch of salt, then mix in the melted margarine. Press the mixture evenly and firmly into the base of a lined 20cm springform cake tin. Place in the fridge to chill.

3. To make the filling, heat the lemon juice with 1 tbsp sweetener in a small pan over a medium heat. When it is hot, take off the heat. Immediately lift the gelatine out of its water and add it to the hot liquid, stirring until dissolved. Leave to cool until barely tepid.

4. In a large bowl, beat together the quark, ricotta, lemon zest, vanilla seeds and remaining sweetener, then whisk in the lemon juice and gelatine mixture.

5. Pour the filling over the biscuit base and smooth the surface. Place in the fridge to set for at least 4 hours, or overnight.

6. To serve, loosen the cheesecake from the tin: if necessary, wave a cook's blowtorch briefly around the outside before releasing the springform clip. Place the cheesecake on a serving plate and top with the strawberries. Cut into slices to serve.

Courgette and cardamom cake

Like the carrots in a carrot cake, courgette keeps this delicious cake lovely and moist. A light cream cheese and lime icing provides a refreshing contrast. The cake will keep in the fridge for a couple of days – just bring it to room temperature before serving to enjoy it at its best.

Serves: 8

Calories: 365 per serving

Sunflower oil spray
250g half-fat margarine
100g caster sugar
4 tbsp granulated sweetener
3 large free-range eggs
250g self-raising flour
1 tsp bicarbonate of soda
1 tsp ground cardamom
1 vanilla pod, split and seeds
    scraped
Finely grated zest of 2 limes
200g courgettes, grated

For the icing
100g icing sugar
1 tbsp light cream cheese
1 tbsp lime juice

To finish
Grated zest of 1 lime

1. Preheat the oven to fan 180°C/gas 4. Spray a 900g (2lb) non-stick loaf tin with a few sprays of oil.

2. Using a stand mixer or electric hand whisk and large bowl, cream together the margarine, caster sugar and sweetener until light and fluffy. Add the eggs, one at a time, beating well after each addition.

3. Sift the flour, bicarbonate of soda and ground cardamom together over the mixture, add the vanilla seeds and lime zest and fold in gently, using a spatula, until just combined. Lastly, fold in the grated courgettes.

4. Spoon the cake mixture into the prepared tin and gently level the surface. Bake on the middle shelf of the oven for 50–60 minutes. To test, insert a skewer into the middle of the cake: it should come out clean; if not give it a little longer.

5. Once cooked, leave the cake to cool in the tin for 5 minutes, then transfer to a wire rack to cool completely.

6. To make the icing, in a bowl, whisk the icing sugar, cream cheese and lime juice together until smoothly combined.

7. Spread the icing on top of the cake and sprinkle with the lime zest. Cut into 8 thick slices to serve.

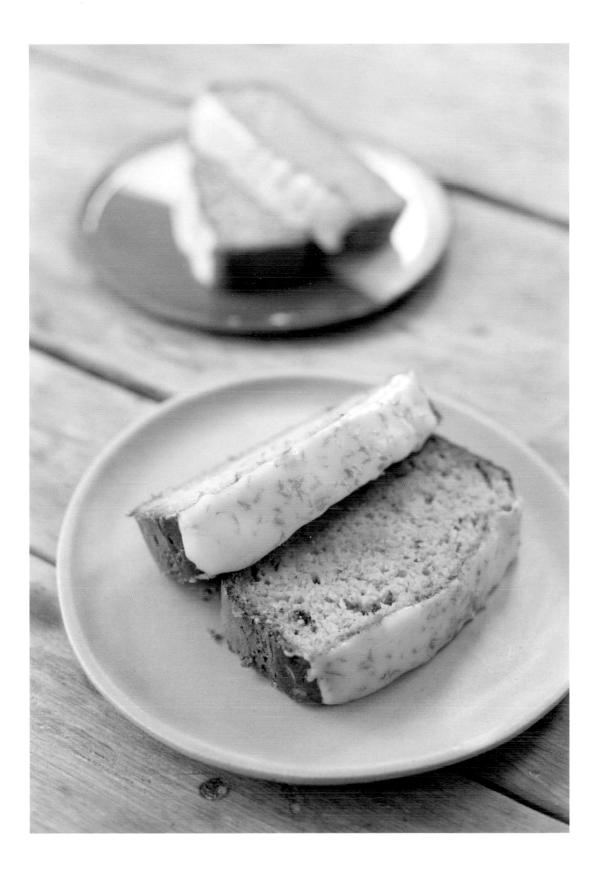

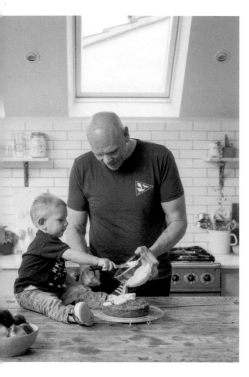

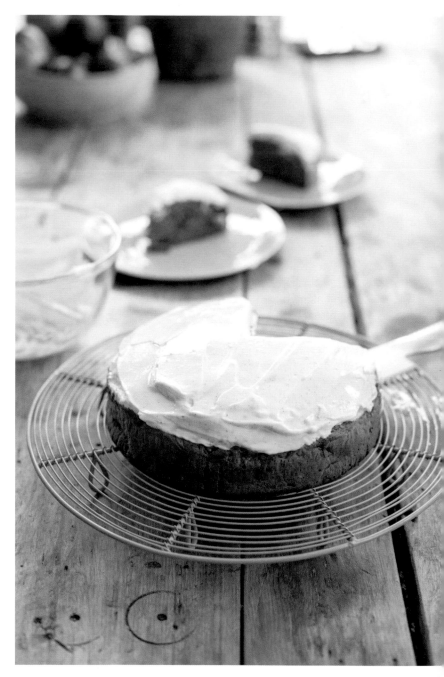

Carrot cake

This delicious cake is packed with extra flavours from the raisins, orange zest, vanilla, cinnamon, nutmeg, pepper and mace. For a lighter, but still creamy, alternative to the traditional full-fat frosting, quark is whipped with vanilla and a little reduced-fat cream cheese. The cake will keep in the fridge for up to 3 days, but bring it to room temperature before serving.

Serves: 8–10

Calories: 270–215 per serving

300g carrots, grated
50g raisins
Finely grated zest of 1 orange
250g self-raising flour
1 tsp bicarbonate of soda
1 tsp baking powder
½ tsp sea salt
2 tsp ground cinnamon
1 tsp freshly grated nutmeg
1 tsp ground mace
½ tsp freshly finely ground
    black pepper
50g butter
25g soft dark brown sugar
4 tsp granulated sweetener
80ml skimmed milk
2 large free-range eggs, beaten
1 vanilla pod, split and seeds
    scraped

For the frosting
150g quark
100g light cream cheese
2–3 tsp granulated sweetener
1 vanilla pod, split and seeds
    scraped

1. Preheat the oven to fan 180°C/gas 4. Line a deep 20cm cake tin with baking parchment.

2. In a large bowl, mix the grated carrots together with the raisins, orange zest, flour, bicarbonate of soda, baking powder, salt and spices, using a wooden spoon.

3. In a small pan over a medium heat, melt the butter with the brown sugar and sweetener. Take the pan off the heat and stir in the milk, then whisk in the beaten eggs and vanilla seeds.

4. Make a well in the middle of the dry ingredients, pour in the egg mixture and stir to combine. Spoon the mixture into the prepared cake tin and bake for 30–35 minutes until cooked. To test, poke a skewer or a knife into the middle: it should come out clean.

5. Leave the cake to cool slightly in the tin for a few minutes, then turn out and place on a wire rack. Leave to cool completely.

6. To make the frosting, whisk the quark, cream cheese, sweetener and vanilla seeds together in a small bowl to combine.

7. Spread the frosting over the top of the cooled cake, using a palette knife. Cut into slices to serve.

Spiced banana and raisin loaf

If you fancy something sweet without the hefty calories of a regular piece of cake, this tasty alternative to banana bread is a great option. Extra banana replaces the usual creamed butter and sugar, and warming spices give it plenty of flavour.

Serves: 8

Calories: 290 per serving

Sunflower oil spray
3 very ripe bananas
   (250g peeled weight)
½ tsp ground cinnamon
½ tsp ground cardamom
1 tsp ground mixed spice
75ml sunflower oil
1 tbsp vanilla extract
3 large free-range eggs, beaten
250g self-raising flour
1 tsp baking powder
1 tsp salt
25g soft light brown sugar
2 tbsp granulated sweetener
40g raisins

1. Preheat the oven to fan 180°C/gas 4. Spray a 900g (2lb) loaf tin with a few sprays of oil.

2. In a bowl, mash the bananas with a fork until smooth. Add the spices, oil, vanilla extract and beaten eggs and mix until evenly combined.

3. In a separate, large bowl, mix together the flour, baking powder, salt, sugar, sweetener and raisins. Pour in the spiced banana mixture and mix until just combined.

4. Pour the mixture into the prepared loaf tin and spread evenly. Bake on the middle shelf of the oven for 35–40 minutes. To test, insert a skewer into the middle of the cake: it should come out clean; if not give it a little longer.

5. Once the tea loaf is cooked, leave it to cool in the tin for 5 minutes, then transfer to a wire rack and allow to cool completely.

6. Cut the tea loaf into 8 thick slices to serve.

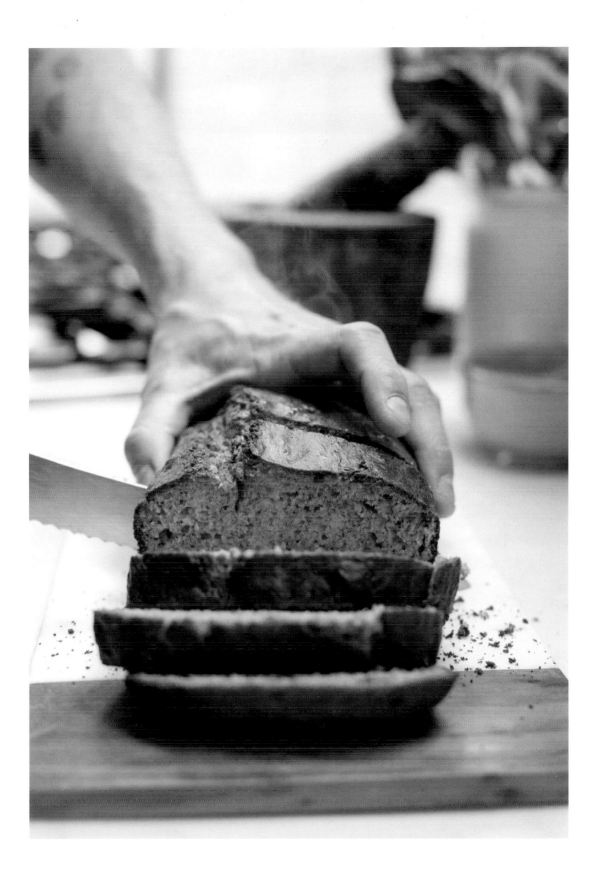

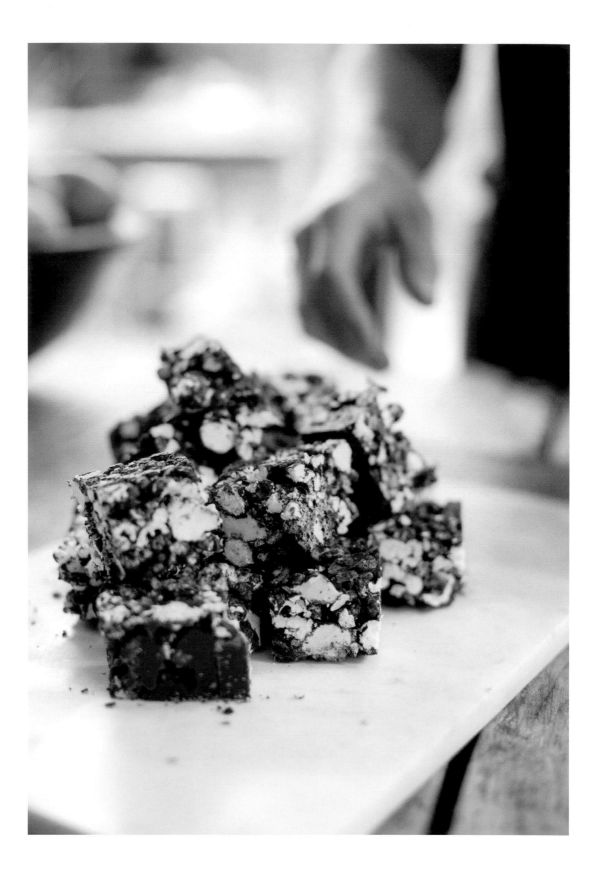

Popcorn bars

Dark chocolate and salted popcorn are strong, intense, contrasting flavours, which work well together in this sweet treat. A good standby to keep in a jar.

Makes: 20

Calories: 90 per bar

200g dark chocolate (70% cocoa solids), broken into pieces
50g puffed rice cereal
40g salted popcorn
50g dried cranberries, halved
50g large marshmallows, quartered

1. Line a 20cm square baking tin with two layers of cling film.

2. Melt the chocolate in a heatproof bowl over a pan of barely simmering water, making sure the bottom of the bowl is not touching the water.

3. Meanwhile, put the cereal, popcorn, cranberries and marshmallows into a bowl and mix well.

4. While the chocolate is still warm, and working quickly, pour it onto the cereal mixture and stir with a rubber spatula until everything is coated.

5. Transfer the mixture to the lined baking tin and press down well. Cover with cling film and place in the fridge to set for a minimum of 2 hours.

6. Turn out onto a board and cut into 20 squares, to enjoy when you get a sweet craving. The bars will keep for up to a week in the fridge.

THE LOWDOWN The percentage on a chocolate bar tells you how much pure cacao is in it. A higher percentage doesn't always guarantee a darker chocolate, but it does guarantee a less sugary one, so if you're watching your sugar intake then go for a chocolate with a higher percentage.

Watermelon ice lollies

On a hot day, what could be more refreshing than these appealing fresh fruit lollies? They are simple to make; you just need an ice-lolly mould and some lolly sticks.

Makes: 8
Calories: 35 per lolly

300g seedless watermelon chunks
100g strawberries, hulled
8 mint leaves
1 tbsp agave
3–4 ripe kiwi fruit, peeled

1. Have ready an 8-mould (each 75ml) ice-lolly tray and 8 wooden ice lolly sticks.

2. Using a jug blender or food processor, blend the watermelon, strawberries, mint and agave together until smooth.

3. Slice 1 kiwi into 8 slices. Lay one slice of kiwi in each ice-lolly mould, pressing it up against the side of the mould. Pour the watermelon purée into the moulds, dividing it evenly and leaving a 1.5cm depth for the kiwi layer (which will be added later).

4. Put the top of the iced lolly mould on and poke a wooden lolly stick into each one. Place in the freezer for 3 hours.

5. Blend the remaining kiwi fruit until smooth – you will need 160g in total.

6. Remove the frozen lollies from the freezer and spoon the kiwi mixture into each mould. Return to the freezer for 2 hours or until completely set.

7. Run a little warm water over the moulds to release the ice lollies. Remove them from the moulds and enjoy.

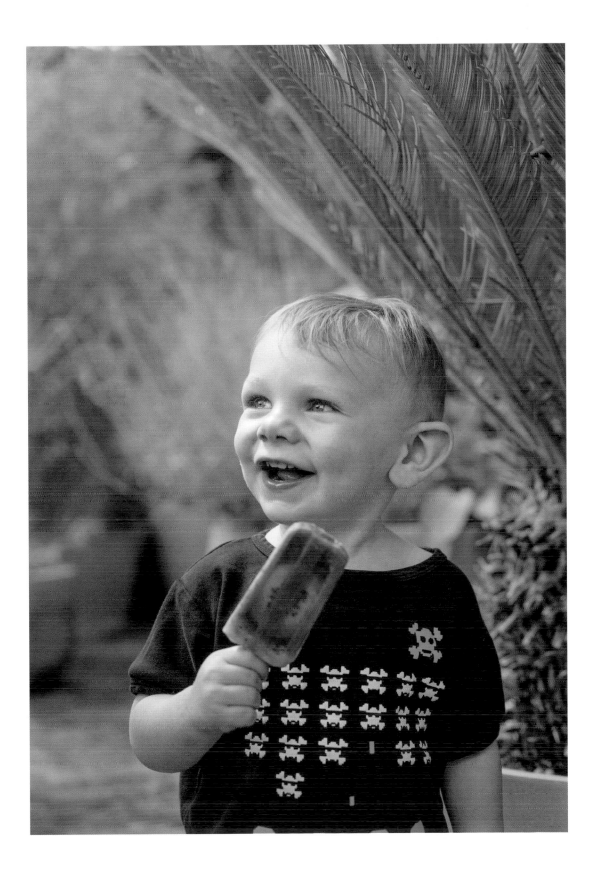

WEIGHING FRESH PRODUCE

The calorie counts for the fruit and vegetables in my recipes are based on the prepared weight, i.e. after any trimming, peeling and coring. You may find the following chart handy when you are calculating your calorie intake for the day, as it tells you how many calories a fruit or vegetable contains once you've prepared it. (You can check the calorie count of most other packaged foods by looking at the nutritional breakdown on the label.)

FRUIT

	Whole weight	Weight after trimming etc.	Calories
Apple, eating (large)	170g	150g	80
Apple, eating (medium)	115g	100g	55
Apple, eating (small)	75g	65g	35
Banana (large)	130g	120g	105
Banana (medium)	110g	100g	85
Banana (small)	90g	80g	70
Blueberries (100g)	100g	100g	45
Bramley apple (large)	240g	210g	85
Raspberries (100g)	100g	100g	35
Strawberries (100g)	100g	100g	40

VEGETABLES

Aubergine (medium)	350g	300g	75
Avocado (medium)	165g	150g	300
Bean sprouts (100g)	100g	100g	35
Broad beans, frozen (100g)	100g	100g	75
Butternut squash (medium)	700g	620g	255
Cabbage, Chinese (100g)	100g	100g	15
Cabbage, red (100g)	100g	100g	25
Cabbage, Savoy (100g)	100g	100g	35
Cabbage, white (100g)	100g	100g	35
Carrot (large)	160g	150g	65
Carrot (medium)	90g	80g	35
Carrot (small)	55g	45g	20
Cauliflower (large)	870g	800g	270
Cauliflower (medium)	625g	575g	195
Cauliflower (small)	290g	265g	125
Celeriac (large)	800g	700g	190
Celeriac (medium)	590g	550g	150
Celeriac (small)	440g	400g	110
Celery stick	30g	30g	5
Chilli, green (medium)	12g	10g	5

Chilli, red (medium)	12g	10g	5	Onion, red (small)	75g	60g	25
Corn-on-the-cob	140g	100g	65	Onions, baby (100g)	100g	100g	40
Corn, baby (100g)	100g	100g	30	Pak choi	110g	100g	20
Courgette (large)	160g	150g	30	Peas, frozen (100g)	100g	100g	95
Courgette (medium)	110g	100g	20	Pepper, green (large)	170g	150g	40
Courgette (small)	70g	60g	10	Pepper, green (medium)	140g	120g	30
Cucumber (large)	400g	390g	60	Pepper, red (large)	170g	150g	40
Cucumber (medium)	300g	290g	45	Pepper, red (medium)	140g	120g	30
Cucumber (small)	150g	140g	25	Pepper, yellow (large)	170g	150g	40
Fennel bulb (large)	250g	230g	70	Pepper, yellow (medium)	140g	120g	30
Fennel bulb (medium)	230g	215g	60	Potato, baking (medium)	250g	250g	210
Fennel bulb (small)	180g	170g	55	Potatoes, new (100g)	100g	100g	75
Green beans (100g)	100g	100g	30	Radishes (100g)	100g	100g	15
Kale (100g)	100g	100g	45	Shallot, banana (large)	70g	60g	15
Kohlrabi (100g)	100g	100g	30	Shallot, banana (medium)	50g	35g	10
Lettuce, iceberg	300g	300g	45	Spring onion	12g	10g	5
Lettuce, little gem	75g	75g	10	Spring onion (bunch of 6)	75g	60g	25
Mangetout (100g)	100g	100g	40	Sweet potato	220g	200g	190
Mushrooms, button (100g)	100g	100g	15	Tenderstem broccoli (100g)	100g	100g	45
Mushrooms, chestnut (100g)	100g	100g	15	Tomato (large)	150g	150g	15
Mushrooms, oyster (100g)	100g	100g	10	Tomato (medium)	85g	85g	15
Onion (large)	240g	220g	90	Tomato (small)	65g	65g	10
Onion (medium)	160g	150g	60	Tomato, beef	200g	200g	35
Onion (small)	75g	60g	25	Tomatoes, cherry (100g)	100g	100g	25
Onion, red (large)	240g	220g	90	Turnips, baby (100g)	100g	100g	30
Onion, red (medium)	160g	150g	60	Watercress (100g)	100g	100g	25

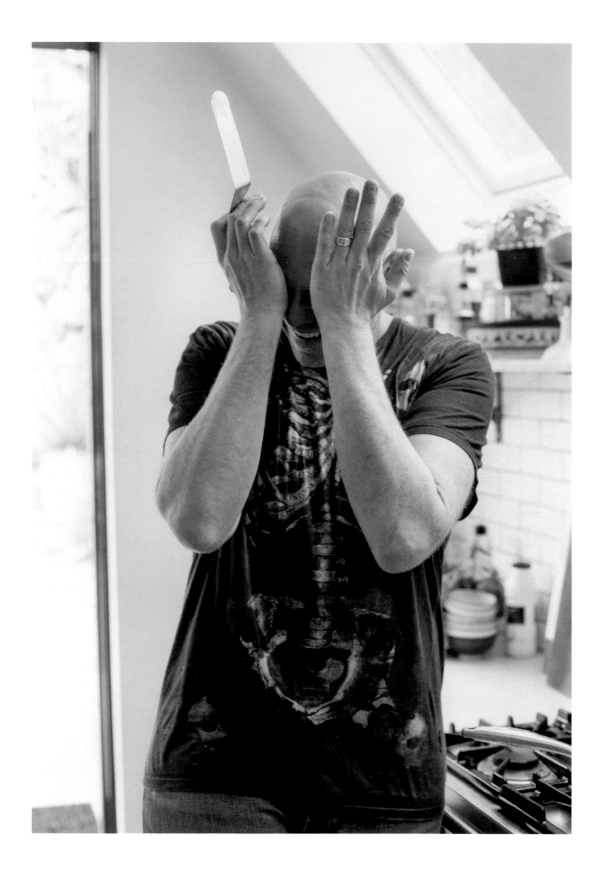

Index

A

anchovies: pea and ham pasta 174
apples: apple and raisin muffins 30
  baked Bramley apples and custard 216
  blueberry and apple Bircher muesli 36
  French apple tarts with mace 220
  spiced red salad 188
apricot and cranberry muffins 40
Asian chicken and pea broth 73
asparagus: creamy mushrooms, poached egg and asparagus 47
aubergines: Japanese miso aubergine 211
  lamb tagine with chickpeas 159
  North African soup 69
avocados: sweet potato and black bean burritos 204–5

B

bacon: chicken casserole 110–11
baking trays 23
bamboo shoots: Asian chicken and pea broth 73
  Thai green chicken curry 125
  Thai red prawn curry 85
bananas: apple and raisin muffins 30
  apricot and cranberry muffins 40
  puffed rice cereal with banana and date yoghurt 39
  spiced banana and raisin loaf 236
barbecue sauce 171
basil: spinach and basil pesto 207
bean sprouts: Asian chicken and pea broth 73
  egg-fried wild rice 212–13
  fish-in-a-bag Chinese style 88
  soy-glazed salmon salad 98
  Thai red prawn curry 85

tom yum soup 65
turkey san choy bow 141
beans (dried) 18
  baked cod with beans, courgettes and chorizo 93
  jerk chicken, cauliflower rice 'n' peas 116
  mixed bean, roasted pepper and feta salad 185
  sweet potato and black bean burritos 204–5
beef: beef stew and dumplings 155
  beef stroganoff 144
  chilli con carne 150–1
  Chinese meatball stir-fry 148–9
  one-layer lasagne 152–3
  pot-roast topside of beef 156–7
  roast beef salad with chimichurri sauce 146
beetroot: pickled beetroot hummus with crudités 180
  spiced red salad 188
  sweet potato and black bean burritos 204–5
berries: frozen red fruit yoghurt and basil 224
  jelly trifle with toasted fennel 223
  overnight porridge with berry compote 35
  see also blueberries etc
Bircher muesli, blueberry and apple 36
biryani, chicken 132–3
biscuits 22
black beans: sweet potato and black bean burritos 204–5
blenders 23
blowtorches 23
blueberries: blueberry and apple Bircher muesli 36
  blueberry, lemon and thyme pancakes 33
breakfast 18–53
broad beans: North African soup 69
  rainbow trout with braised fennel 91
broccoli: chicken saltimbocca 108–9

fish-in-a-bag Chinese style 88
South Indian fish curry 82
broths: Asian chicken and pea broth 73
  salad broth 56
burgers, spicy Moroccan lamb 165
burritos, sweet potato and black bean 204–5
butter beans: baked cod with beans, courgettes and chorizo 93
butternut squash soup, Thai-style 66

C

cabbage: coleslaw 120
  slaw 171
  toasted cabbage tart with ricotta and lemon 200
  turkey ragu with white cabbage linguine 130
Cajun prawn and kale salad 102
cakes: carrot cake 235
  courgette and cardamom cake 232
  spiced banana and raisin loaf 236
calorie-restricted diets 8–10
carbohydrates 8
carrots: beef stew and dumplings 155
  carrot cake 235
  chicken biryani 132–3
  chicken casserole 110–11
  Chinese meatball stir-fry 148–9
  coleslaw 120
  pot-roast topside of beef 156–7
  salad broth 56
  soy-glazed salmon salad 98
  spicy Moroccan lamb burgers 165
  sweet potato and black bean burritos 204–5
  turkey ragu with white cabbage linguine 130
  veg and lentil soup 74
cauliflower: cauliflower 'rice' 18, 179

chicken biryani 132–3
jerk chicken, cauliflower rice 'n' peas 116
spicy lamb mince curry 160
stuffed peppers 196
celeriac: celeriac mash 112
cream of celeriac soup with truffle oil 62
celery: pot-roast topside of beef 156–7
veg and lentil soup 74
cheese 19
chicken with tomato, mascarpone and basil 119
chilli con carne 150–1
easy pizza with Parma ham and mozzarella 177
Greek kebabs 115
griddled veg and halloumi with couscous 186
Mediterranean puff pastry tart 208
mixed bean, roasted pepper and feta salad 185
one-layer lasagne 152–3
salmon, egg and feta 'muffins' 53
shakshuka breakfast eggs 44
spinach and paneer curry 203
stuffed peppers 196
turkey and courgette burgers with mozzarella 120–1
see also ricotta
cheesecake: tropical cheesecake pots 228
vanilla and strawberry cheesecake 231
chicken 12, 18, 104–41
Asian chicken and pea broth 73
chicken and mushroom filo crunch 128–9
chicken and sweetcorn soup 70
chicken biryani 132–3
chicken casserole 110–11
chicken saltimbocca 108–9
chicken satay 126
chicken tikka masala 122–3
chicken with fennel, garlic and tomatoes 138

chicken with peas, mushrooms and celeriac mash 112
chicken with tomato, mascarpone and basil 119
Greek kebabs 115
jerk chicken and tomato salad 106
jerk chicken, cauliflower rice 'n' peas 116
piri piri chicken 136–7
poaching a chicken crown 105
Southern-style chicken 134–5
Thai green chicken curry 125
tom yum soup 65
chickpeas 18
baked falafel with tzatziki 191
chickpea and spinach curry 192
lamb tagine with chickpeas 159
North African soup 69
pickled beetroot hummus 180
chillies 18
Asian chicken and pea broth 73
chicken satay 126
chickpea and spinach curry 192
chilli con carne 150–1
chimichurri sauce 146
fish-in-a-bag Chinese style 88
lamb doner 162–3
piri piri chicken 136–7
pork samosa pie 168
spicy lamb mince curry 160
tom yum soup 65
turkey san choy bow 141
chimichurri sauce 146
Chinese cabbage: soy-glazed salmon salad 98
Chinese meatball stir-fry 148–9
chipotle yoghurt 204
chocolate: coffee and chocolate custard pots 227
popcorn bars 239
chorizo: baked cod with beans, courgettes and chorizo 93
citrus dressing, lettuce with 152–3

coconut milk: Asian chicken and pea broth 73
prawn curry with peas 78
South Indian fish curry 82
Thai green chicken curry 125
Thai red prawn curry 85
Thai-style butternut squash soup 66
cod: baked cod with beans, courgettes and chorizo 93
Italian seafood pot 94
South Indian fish curry 82
coffee and chocolate custard pots 227
coleslaw 120
containers 15, 25
corn (baby): Thai red prawn curry 85
tom yum soup 65
cornflour 18
courgettes: baked cod with beans, courgettes and chorizo 93
courgette and cardamom cake 232
courgette and ricotta pancakes 198
creamy wild mushroom courgetti 195
Italian seafood pot 94
lamb tagine with chickpeas 159
Mediterranean puff pastry tart 208
North African soup 69
one-layer lasagne 152–3
Provençal salmon traybake 87
smoked ham and courgette tortilla 51
spicy Moroccan lamb burgers 165
spinach and basil pesto courgetti 207
Thai green chicken curry 125
turkey and courgette burgers with mozzarella 120–1
couscous, griddled veg and halloumi with 186
cranberries: apricot and cranberry muffins 40
popcorn bars 239
cranberry juice: jelly trifle 223

246

cream alternatives 18
cream cheese: carrot cake 235
    tropical cheesecake pots 228
crumbles: beef crumble 146
    chicken crumble 110–11
cucumber: jerk chicken and
    tomato salad 106
    katchumber salad 123
    soy-glazed salmon salad 98
    tzatziki 191
curry: Asian chicken and pea
    broth 73
    chicken biryani 132–3
    chicken tikka masala 122–3
    chickpea and spinach curry
    192
    pork samosa pie 168
    prawn curry with peas 78
    South Indian fish curry 82
    spicy lamb mince curry 160
    spinach and paneer curry 203
    Thai green chicken curry 125
    Thai red prawn curry 85
    Thai-style butternut squash
    soup 66
custard: baked Bramley apples
    and custard 216
    coffee and chocolate custard
    pots 227
    jelly trifle with toasted fennel
    223

D
dairy products 19
dates: puffed rice cereal with
    banana and date yoghurt 39
doughnuts with sweet five-spice
    dust 42
dressings 12–13
dumplings 155

E
eggs 19
    creamy mushrooms, poached
    egg and asparagus 47
    egg-fried wild rice 212–13
    salmon, egg and feta 'muffins'
    53
    scrambled Cajun eggs with
    spinach and kale 48
    shakshuka breakfast eggs 44

smoked ham and courgette
    tortilla 51
tuna niçoise 101
equipment 23–5

F
falafel with tzatziki 191
fennel: chicken with fennel,
    garlic and tomatoes 138
    Italian seafood pot 94
    rainbow trout with braised
    fennel 91
    spiced red salad 188
feta see cheese
filo pastry: chicken and
    mushroom filo crunch 128–9
    pork samosa pie 168
fish and seafood 19, 76–103
    baked tuna fish cakes 97
    fish-in-a-bag Chinese style
    88–9
    see also cod, salmon etc
food processors 23
French apple tarts with mace
    220
frozen red fruit yoghurt and basil
    224
fruit 19
    see also apples, berries,
    strawberries etc

G
garlic 18
ginger 18
goat's cheese: Mediterranean
    puff pastry tart 208
graters 23
Greek kebabs 115
green beans: chicken biryani
    132–3
    mixed bean, roasted pepper
    and feta salad 185
    Provençal salmon traybake 87
    Thai green chicken curry 125
    tuna niçoise 101
griddle pans 23

H
halloumi: griddled veg and
    halloumi with couscous 186
ham: chicken saltimbocca 108–9

easy pizza with Parma ham
    and mozzarella 177
    pea and ham pasta 174
    smoked ham and courgette
    tortilla 51
harissa yoghurt 165
herb dressing 186
herbs 19
hot sauce 19
hummus, pickled beetroot 180

I
ice lollies, watermelon 240
ingredients 18–22
Italian seafood pot 94

J
Japanese miso aubergine 211
jelly trifle with toasted fennel 223
jerk chicken and tomato salad
    106
jerk chicken, cauliflower rice 'n'
    peas 116

K
kale: Cajun prawn and kale
    salad 102
    pot-roast topside of beef
    156–7
    scrambled Cajun eggs with
    spinach and kale 48
katchumber salad 123
kebabs, Greek 115
kidney beans: jerk chicken,
    cauliflower rice 'n' peas 116
kiwi fruit: watermelon ice lollies
    240
kohlrabi: soy-glazed salmon
    salad 98

L
lamb: lamb doner 162–3
    lamb tagine with chickpeas
    159
    spicy lamb mince curry 160
    spicy Moroccan lamb burgers
    165
lasagne, one-layer 152–3
lentils: spicy lamb mince curry
    160
    veg and lentil soup 74

lettuce: lettuce with citrus
dressing 152–3
pulled pork tacos 172–3
roast beef salad 146
salad broth 56
sweet potato and black bean
burritos 204–5
tuna niçoise 101
turkey san choy bow 141

M

mangetout: Asian chicken and
pea broth 73
Thai red prawn curry 85
tom yum soup 65
mangoes: tropical cheesecake
pots 228
marshmallows: popcorn bars 239
mayo, yuzu 81
meat 20, 142–77
see also beef, lamb etc
meat thermometers 25
meatball stir-fry, Chinese 148–9
Mediterranean puff pastry tart
208
milk 19
rice pudding with rosewater
and raspberries 219
miso aubergine, Japanese 211
mixed bean, roasted pepper and
feta salad 185
Moroccan lamb burgers 165
motivation 14–15
mozzarella see cheese
muesli, blueberry and apple 36
muffin trays 25
muffins: apple and raisin
muffins 30
apricot and cranberry muffins
40
salmon, egg and feta 'muffins'
53
mushrooms: beef stew and
dumplings 155
beef stroganoff 144
chicken and mushroom filo
crunch 128–9
chicken casserole 110–11
chicken with peas,
mushrooms and celeriac
mash 112

Chinese meatball stir-fry
148–9
creamy mushrooms, poached
egg and asparagus 47
creamy wild mushroom
courgetti 195
egg-fried wild rice 212–13
one-layer lasagne 152–3
stuffed peppers 196
tom yum soup 65
turkey san choy bow 141
mustard 19

N

non-stick pans 25
noodles: Asian chicken and pea
broth 73
North African soup 69

O

oats: overnight porridge 35
oil, spray 10–12, 20
olives: baked cod with beans,
courgettes and chorizo 93
Italian seafood pot 94
mixed bean, roasted pepper
and feta salad 185
Provençal salmon traybake 87
stuffed peppers 196
one-layer lasagne 152–3
onions: chicken and sweetcorn
soup 70
chicken biryani 132–3
chicken casserole 110–11
chicken tikka masala 122–3
chicken with fennel, garlic and
tomatoes 138
cream of celeriac soup 62
cream of tomato soup 61
Italian seafood pot 94
North African soup 69
pea and mint soup 58
pickled pink onions 172–3
pork samosa pie 168
pot-roast topside of beef
156–7
Provençal salmon traybake 87
South Indian fish curry 82
Thai green chicken curry 125
turkey ragu 130
veg and lentil soup 74

oranges: pulled pork tacos
172–3
spiced red salad 188
orzo pasta: Italian seafood pot 94
oven thermometers 25
overnight porridge 35

P

pak choi: fish-in-a-bag Chinese
style 88
pork tenderloin with Japanese
ponzu dressing 166
pancakes: blueberry, lemon and
thyme pancakes 33
courgette and ricotta
pancakes 198
paneer: spinach and paneer
curry 203
Parma ham see ham
passion fruit: tropical
cheesecake pots 228
pasta: Italian seafood pot 94
pea and ham pasta 174
pastry 20
see also filo pastry; tarts
peanut butter: chicken satay 126
peas: Asian chicken and pea
broth 73
chicken with peas,
mushrooms and celeriac
mash 112
egg-fried wild rice 212–13
pea and ham pasta 174
pea and mint soup 58
pork samosa pie 168
prawn curry with peas 78
rainbow trout with braised
fennel 91
salmon, egg and feta 'muffins'
53
smoked ham and courgette
tortilla 51
South Indian fish curry 82
spicy lamb mince curry 160
pepper 20
peppers: Cajun prawn and kale
salad 102
chicken tikka masala 122–3
Chinese meatball stir-fry
148–9
egg-fried wild rice 212–13

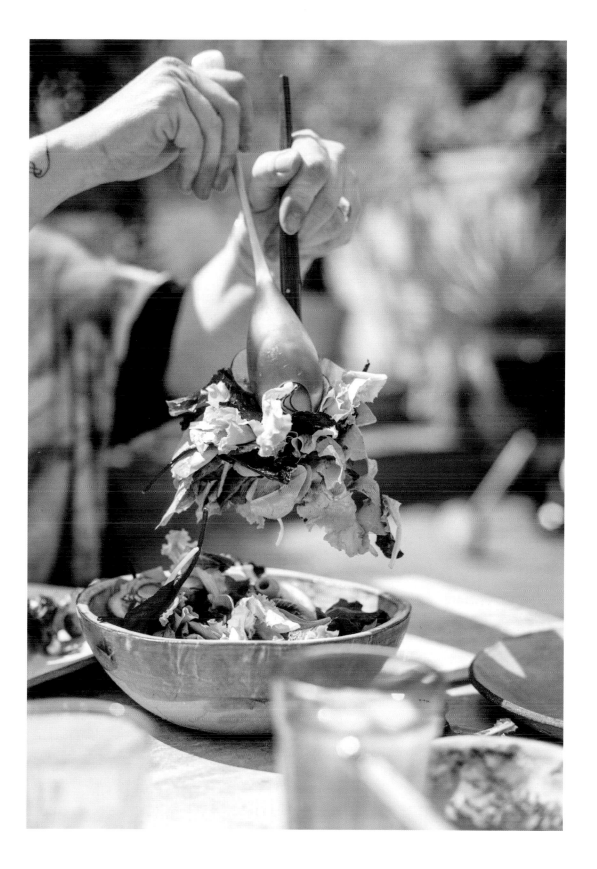

Greek kebabs 115
griddled veg and halloumi with
couscous 186
jerk chicken, cauliflower rice
'n' peas 116
Mediterranean puff pastry tart
208
mixed bean, roasted pepper
and feta salad 185
piri piri chicken 136–7
Provençal salmon traybake 87
scrambled Cajun eggs with
spinach and kale 48
shakshuka breakfast eggs 44
stuffed peppers 196
Thai green chicken curry 125
Thai red prawn curry 85
pesto, spinach and basil 207
pickled beetroot hummus 180
pickled pink onions 172–3
pickled radishes 136–7
pineapple: tropical cheesecake
pots 228
piri piri chicken 136–7
pizza with Parma ham and
mozzarella 177
poaching a chicken crown 105
ponzu dressing 166
popcorn bars 239
pork: pork samosa pie 168
pork tenderloin with Japanese
ponzu dressing 166
pulled pork tacos 172–3
sticky pork chops 171
porridge, overnight 35
pot-roast topside of beef 156–7
potatoes: baked tuna fish cakes
97
herby potato salad 134–5
pork samosa pie 168
salad broth 56
tuna niçoise 101
prawns: Cajun prawn and kale
salad 102
Italian seafood pot 94
prawn curry with peas 78
Thai red prawn curry 85
tom yum soup 65
Provençal salmon traybake 87
puffed rice cereal: popcorn bars
239

puffed rice with banana and
date yoghurt 39
pulled pork tacos 172–3

Q
quark 19
carrot cake 235

R
radishes, pickled 136–7
ragu, turkey 130
rainbow trout with braised
fennel 91
raisins: apple and raisin muffins
30
carrot cake 235
spiced banana and raisin
loaf 236
raspberries, rice pudding with
219
red cabbage: coleslaw 120
slaw 171
spiced red salad 188
restaurants 16
rice: chicken biryani 132–3
chicken tikka masala 122–3
egg-fried wild rice 212–13
fish-in-a-bag Chinese style 88
prawn curry with peas 78
rice pudding with rosewater
and raspberries 219
spicy lamb mince curry 160
ricotta 231
blueberry, lemon and thyme
pancakes 33
courgette and ricotta
pancakes 198
one-layer lasagne 152–3
toasted cabbage tart with
ricotta and lemon 200
tomato, ricotta and basil salad
183

S
salad broth 56
salads: Cajun prawn and kale
salad 102
coleslaw 120
herby potato salad 134–5
jerk chicken and tomato
salad 106

katchumber salad 123
mixed bean, roasted pepper
and feta salad 185
roast beef salad 146
slaw 171
soy-glazed salmon salad 98
spiced red salad 188
tomato, ricotta and basil
salad 183
tuna niçoise 101
salmon: Provençal salmon
traybake 87
salmon, egg and feta 'muffins'
53
soy-glazed salmon salad 98
salt 20
salt and pepper squid 81
satay, chicken 126
scrambled Cajun eggs 48
sea bass: fish-in-a-bag Chinese
style 88–9
seafood and fish 19, 76–103
shakshuka breakfast eggs 44
slaw 171
smoked cod: Italian seafood pot
94
smoked ham and courgette
tortilla 51
smoked paprika dressing 183
smoked salmon: salmon, egg
and feta 'muffins' 53
snacking 15–16, 22
soups 54–75
Asian chicken and pea broth
73
chicken and sweetcorn soup
70
cream of celeriac soup 62
cream of tomato soup 61
North African soup 69
pea and mint soup 58
salad broth 56
Thai-style butternut squash
soup 66
tom yum soup 65
veg and lentil soup 74
South Indian fish curry 82
Southern-style chicken 134–5
soy sauce: fish-in-a-bag Chinese
style 88
soy-glazed salmon salad 98

spices 20
spinach: Asian chicken and pea
    broth 73
    chickpea and spinach curry
        192
    prawn curry with peas 78
    scrambled Cajun eggs with
        spinach and kale 48
    spinach and basil pesto
        courgetti 207
    spinach and paneer curry 203
spiralisers 25, 179
spray oil 10–12, 20
spring onions: Asian chicken
    and pea broth 73
squid, salt and pepper 81
stews: beef stew and dumplings
    155
    beef stroganoff 144
    chicken casserole 110–11
    turkey ragu 130
sticky pork chops 171
stir-fry, Chinese meatball 148–9
stock 20–2
strawberries: vanilla and
    strawberry cheesecake 231
    watermelon ice lollies 240
sweet potato and black bean
    burritos 204–5
sweetcorn: chicken and
    sweetcorn soup 70
    egg-fried wild rice 212–13
sweeteners 22

T
tacos, pulled pork 172–3
tagine: lamb with chickpeas 159
tarts: French apple tarts with
    mace 220
    Mediterranean puff pastry
        tart 208
    toasted cabbage tart with
        ricotta and lemon 200
Thai green chicken curry 125
Thai red prawn curry 85
Thai-style butternut squash
    soup 66
thermometers 25
tiger prawns see prawns
tikka masala, chicken 122–3
tom yum soup 65

tomatoes: baked cod with beans,
    courgettes and chorizo 93
    chicken biryani 132–3
    chicken tikka masala 122–3
    chicken with fennel, garlic and
        tomatoes 138
    chicken with tomato,
        mascarpone and basil 119
    chickpea and spinach curry
        192
    chilli con carne 150–1
    cream of tomato soup 61
    easy pizza with Parma ham
        and mozzarella 177
    Italian seafood pot 94
    jerk chicken and tomato
        salad 106
    jerk chicken, cauliflower rice
        'n' peas 116
    katchumber salad 123
    lamb tagine with chickpeas
        159
    North African soup 69
    one-layer lasagne 152–3
    prawn curry with peas 78
    Provençal salmon traybake 87
    pulled pork tacos 172–3
    roast beef salad 146
    shakshuka breakfast eggs 44
    South Indian fish curry 82
    spinach and basil pesto
        courgetti 207
    tomato, ricotta and basil
        salad 183
    turkey ragu with white
        cabbage linguine 130
tortilla, smoked ham and
    courgette 51
tortillas 22
    easy pizza with Parma ham
        and mozzarella 177
    lamb doner 162–3
    pulled pork tacos 172–3
    sweet potato and black bean
        burritos 204–5
    tortilla chips 150–1
trifle, jelly 223
tropical cheesecake pots 228
trout with braised fennel 91
tuna: baked tuna fish cakes 97
    tuna niçoise 101

turkey 22
    turkey and courgette burgers
        with mozzarella 120–1
    turkey ragu with white
        cabbage linguine 130
    turkey san choy bow 141
turnips: beef stew and
    dumplings 155
tzatziki 191

V
vanilla and strawberry
    cheesecake 231
vegetables 22, 178–213
    griddled veg and halloumi with
        couscous 186
    pickled beetroot hummus with
        crudités 180
    veg and lentil soup 74
    see also peppers, tomatoes etc

W
water chestnuts: turkey san choy
    bow 141
watercress: roast beef salad
    146
    salad broth 56
watermelon ice lollies 240
wild rice, egg-fried 212–13
wine: chicken casserole 110–11
    turkey ragu 130

Y
yellow split peas: pea and mint
    soup 58
yoghurt 19
    blueberry and apple Bircher
        muesli 36
    chicken tikka masala 122–3
    chipotle yoghurt 204
    coleslaw 120
    flavoured yoghurt 220
    frozen red fruit yoghurt and
        basil 224
    harissa yoghurt 165
    lamb doner 162–3
    puffed rice cereal with banana
        and date yoghurt 39
    tropical cheesecake pots 228
    tzatziki 191
yuzu mayo 81

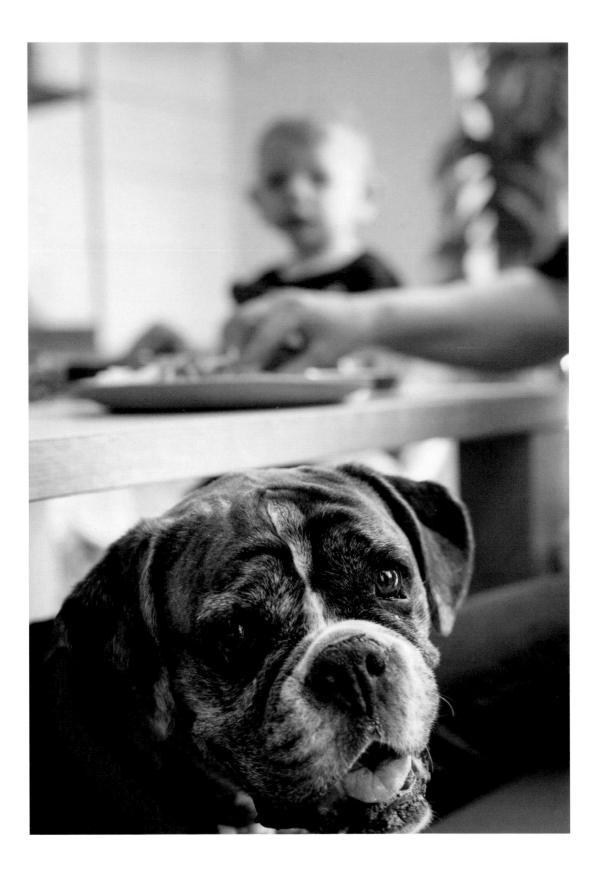

Shout outs and thanks!

Firstly and most importantly, I'm grateful for the support I get from home. Beth, Acey, the dogs and crew (Suze and Katie) – thank you so much for allowing me to just get on with doing stuff. Without you making sure that everything is in the right place and looked after, I wouldn't have the headspace for writing a book.

Thank you to everyone at Bloomsbury and Absolute who has been involved in creating yet another amazing, incredible book. Your help and vision makes my life so much easier. Lisa Pendreigh, Xa Shaw Stewart, Jon Croft, Natalie Bellos, Richard Atkinson, Ellen Williams and Arlene Alexander, all of you guys are by far the best team of publishers and I'm so proud to work with you lot. Nigel Newton, thank you so much for your belief; hopefully we can pop out for another lunch date soon!

To the Marlow squad – the whole team at The Hand & Flowers and The Coach: you are the foundation that everything is built on and your drive for maintaining those high standards on a daily basis is what allows me to put pen to paper, take photographs or just cook the recipes that will end up in a book. Thank you so much for making those places work without the need for me being there.

To the ever-dependable Alex Longstaff, you are the most patient person and put up with my easily distracted, completely childish, and very often stupid behaviour. Thank you so much for helping me focus and actually get the words typed.

To the team at Bone Soup who helped to create a brilliant television show driven by emotion and heartfelt stories, showcasing the beautiful food that's also in this great book. Richard Bowron, Sarah Myland, Madeline Eaton, Georgia Mills, Sophie Wells, Ceri Elms, Richard Hill, Jack Coathupe, Robbie Johnson, David Calvert, Joanna Boyle, Maria Dennett, Joe Panayiotou, Nick Murray, Tom Berrow, Chris Mallet, Dan Blackman, Lucy Kattenhorn and Martin Morrison, you guys are such a joy to work with.

Thank you to David Eldridge at Two Associates for the beautiful design of this book, and to Janet Illsley as the project editor, Jen Hopley for analysing (and generally being great) and Laura Herring for giving me extra vocabulary – excellent work guys, very proud!

Cristian and Bríd, I love working with you guys so much. The vision and the aesthetic of your pictures is always so beautiful, no matter what I throw at you. Cristian, you are a wizard!

The prop styling and art direction of this book are another thing of beauty. The photographs feel full of life and 'at home', and for that I have to thank Lydia McPherson and Lauren Miller. Once again, you have created a fantastic space to shoot in. This leads me to thank John and Lisa at E4 Kitchen Location for the use of their home and for allowing us to make a mess of it every day for two weeks; love you guys.

Now for the most important job of the lot – the food stylists. Nicole Herft, Chris Mackett, Holly Cochrane, Rosie Mackean and Emma Laws, thanks for coming with me on the journey towards easy, lower calorie cooking that tastes great. Nicole, you are a rude, loud and boisterous Australian and I love you dearly. Thank you so much for helping to make this brilliant book come to life, and for holding my hand through the development of the television series.

Borra Garson – ta mate! Keep guiding us through the whirlwind of life. I listen to everything you say and take it on board, even when it doesn't look like it!

Lastly, to an inspirational team of dieters. Anybody wanting to lose weight just needs to look at what you have achieved. I am so proud of every single one of you. Your stories show to millions of people what can be done with some hard work and enthusiasm. Kayleigh Daniel, Özgür 'Ozi' Maden, Pittri Magnusen, Andrew Grant, Louise Fraser, David Shepherd, Ki Price, Samantha Goodman, Rev. Jenny Ellis, Leigh-Jayne Smith, Sandra Fontaine, Beth Meeks and Tom Mitchell: love you all very much.

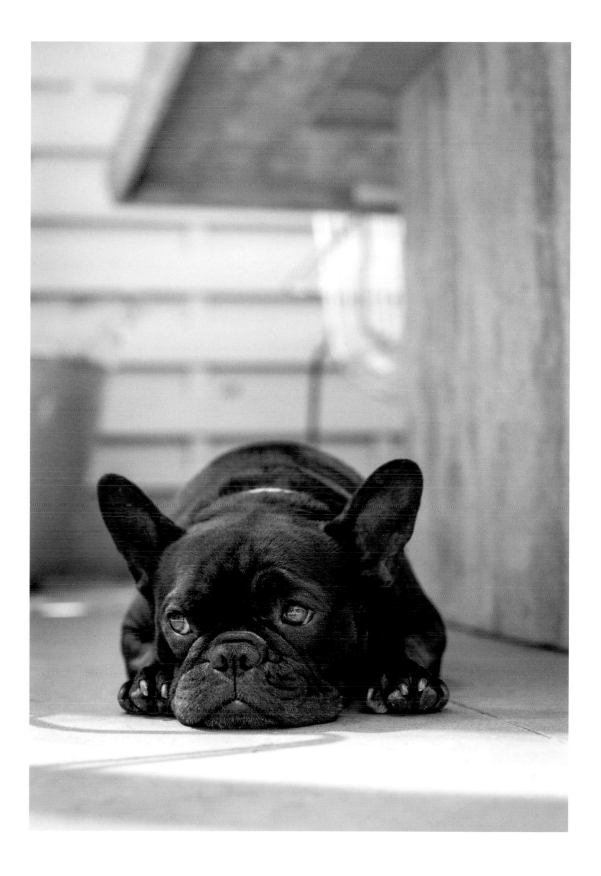

Absolute Press
An imprint of Bloomsbury Publishing Plc

50 Bedford Square
London
WC1B 3DP
UK

www.bloomsbury.com

ABSOLUTE PRESS and the A. logo are trademarks
of Bloomsbury Publishing Plc

First published in Great Britain 2017

British Library Cataloguing-in-Publication Data
A catalogue record for this book is available from the
British Library.

ISBN: HB: 978-1-4729-4929-5
         ePub: 978-1-4729-4930-1

10 9 8 7 6 5 4 3

Project Edit: Janet Illsley
Design: Two Associates
Photographs: Cristian Barnett, crisbarnett.com
Food Styling: Tom Kerridge, Nicole Herft and
    Chris Mackett
Art Direction and Styling: Lydia McPherson
Illustrations: Two Associates
Index: Hilary Bird

Printed and bound by Bell and Bain Ltd, Glasgow

To find out more about our authors and books visit
www.bloomsbury.com. Here you will find extracts,
author interviews, details of forthcoming events and
the option to sign up for our newsletters.

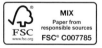